Securing and Excelling in a **Pharmacy Residency**

Edited by

Michael A. Crouch, PharmD, FASHP, BCPS (AQ Cardiology)

Professor and Associate Dean for
Academic Affairs and Professional Education
Director, Teaching and Learning Certificate Program
Clinical Specialist, Cardiology
Bill Gatton College of Pharmacy
East Tennessee State University
Johnson City, Tennessee

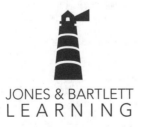

JONES & BARTLETT
LEARNING

World Headquarters
Jones & Bartlett Learning
5 Wall Street
Burlington, MA 01803
978-443-5000
info@jblearning.com
www.jblearning.com

Jones & Bartlett Learning books and products are available through most bookstores and online booksellers. To contact Jones & Bartlett Learning directly, call 800-832-0034, fax 978-443-8000, or visit our website, www.jblearning.com.

The authors, editor, and publisher have made every effort to provide accurate information. However, they are not responsible for errors, omissions, or for any outcomes related to the use of the contents of this book and take no responsibility for the use of the products and procedures described. Treatments and side effects described in this book may not be applicable to all people; likewise, some people may require a dose or experience a side effect that is not described herein. Drugs and medical devices are discussed that may have limited availability controlled by the Food and Drug Administration (FDA) for use only in a research study or clinical trial. Research, clinical practice, and government regulations often change the accepted standard in this field. When consideration is being given to use of any drug in the clinical setting, the healthcare provider or reader is responsible for determining FDA status of the drug, reading the package insert, and reviewing prescribing information for the most up-to-date recommendations on dose, precautions, and contraindications, and determining the appropriate usage for the product. This is especially important in the case of drugs that are new or seldom used.

Production Credits

Publisher: David D. Cella
Acquisitions Editor: Katey Birtcher
Managing Editor: Maro Gartside
Associate Production Editor: Jill Morton
Marketing Manager: Grace Richards
Manufacturing and Inventory Control Supervisor:
  Amy Bacus

Composition: Cenveo
Cover Design: Scott Moden
Cover Image: © photoslb com/ShutterStock, Inc.
Printing and Binding: Malloy Incorporated
Cover Printing: Malloy Incorporated

Some images in this book feature models. These models do not necessarily endorse, represent, or participate in the activities represented in the images.

Library of Congress Cataloging-in-Publication Data
Securing and excelling in a pharmacy residency / [edited] by Michael A. Crouch.
    p.; cm.
  Includes bibliographical references and index.
  ISBN-13: 978-1-4496-0483-7
  ISBN-10: 1-4496-0483-8
  I. Crouch, Michael A. (Michael Andrew), 1969-
  [DNLM: 1. Education, Pharmacy, Continuing. 2. Internship and Residency. QV 20]
  LC classification not assigned
  615.1071'55—dc23
                    2011033113

6048
Printed in the United States of America
15 14 13 12 11   10 9 8 7 6 5 4 3 2 1

To Candace, Jack, Julia, and Anna

for their never-ending support . . .

CONTENTS

PREFACE

Students frequently ask, "Should I do a residency?" and if so, "What do I need to do to get one?" Today, these questions are more relevant than ever. The American Society of Health-System Pharmacists (ASHP) and the American College of Clinical Pharmacy have adopted the stance that by the year 2020 the completion of an ASHP-accredited residency should be a requirement for all new college of pharmacy graduates who will be providing direct patient care. Although the 2020 initiative is a significant step forward for the profession, it furthers the competitive nature of pharmacy residencies and compounds an already existing shortage of available positions.

Colleges and schools of pharmacy advise students regarding residency training by means of lectures, seminars, elective courses, and unique curricular tracks. ASHP, the accrediting body for pharmacy residencies, supplies information about residency training through its website and official journal, the *American Journal of Health-System Pharmacists*. Other professional organizations, including the American College of Clinical Pharmacy, the American Pharmacists Association, and the Academy of Managed Care Pharmacy, also offer a variety of resources related to postgraduate training. Although these organizations provide vital information related to postgraduate residencies, it is somewhat difficult to retrieve and assimilate.

Securing and Excelling in a Pharmacy Residency primarily aims to serve as a comprehensive and convenient guide to individuals seeking a pharmacy residency. The first section of the book reviews the case for pharmacy residencies, and it contains eight chapters that introduce the reader to numerous postgraduate training opportunities. The second section of the book tackles finding the right residency. It begins with a checklist and key websites related to obtaining a pharmacy residency, followed by eight chapters that offer guidance regarding being a stronger applicant, beginning the search, the application and interview process, and steps to select a residency.

A secondary aim of *Securing and Excelling in a Pharmacy Residency* is to guide individuals currently enrolled in a residency, and their mentors, to excel during the program. As such, the book includes a third section that speaks to making the most of a residency. It provides a checklist and key readings related to excelling in a pharmacy residency, followed by seven chapters that present an overview of the year, general guidance to be successful, and typical resident responsibilities in the areas of service, teaching, and scholarship. The final chapter of the book addresses options after residency training, which should be of great interest to both current residents and their advisers.

This book would not be possible without the considerable work of the section editors and chapter contributors. These include individuals from nationally known residency programs, including the Universities of North Carolina, Kentucky, and Arizona, as well as the Medical University of South Carolina, Virginia Commonwealth University, Temple University, and Duke University Medical Center. It also has contributors from emerging residency programs, such as East Tennessee State University, among others. I sincerely thank the contributors for their work that made this reference a reality.

Regardless of your reason to open this book, I hope you find it a practical guide. It aspires to serve as a handbook for student pharmacists seeking a residency as well as their faculty mentors. It also aims to be a reference for current residents and residency program leaders. The main goal of the book is to encourage high-quality pharmacy residency training, which elevates the profession and ultimately patient care.

ABOUT THE EDITOR

MICHAEL A. CROUCH is professor and associate dean for academic affairs and professional education at the Bill Gatton College of Pharmacy, East Tennessee State University (ETSU). In addition to his administrative appointment at ETSU, he directs the college's Teaching and Learning Certificate program. Previous leadership roles related to pharmacy residency training include residency program director for internal medicine, and later cardiology, at Virginia Commonwealth University, and residency program coordinator at South University.

Dr. Crouch attended the University of North Carolina where he received a bachelor of science in pharmacy in 1992. He pursued additional training at the Medical University of South Carolina, receiving a doctor of pharmacy degree in 1995. His postgraduate training entailed a first-year residency at Wake Forest University Baptist Medical Center (1992–1993) and a second-year residency, with emphasis in cardiology, at the Medical University of South Carolina (1995–1996).

Dr. Crouch is a board certified pharmacotherapy specialist who also holds added qualifications in cardiology. He is an active member of the American Society of Health-System Pharmacists, which named him a fellow in 2009, and the American Association of Colleges of Pharmacy and the American College of Clinical Pharmacy. Dr. Crouch publishes broadly in his areas of expertise, including research related to cardiovascular pharmacotherapeutics and the scholarship of teaching. He serves on the cardiology editorial advisory board for the *Annals of Pharmacotherapy* and edited another book titled *Cardiovascular Pharmacotherapy: A Point-of-Care Guide.*

Ray R. Maddox, PharmD, FASHP
Director, Clinical Pharmacy, Research, and Pulmonary Medicine
St. Joseph's/Candler Health System
Savannah, Georgia

Dominic P. Ragucci, PharmD, BCPS
Clinical Assistant Professor
PGY1 Residency Program Director
South Carolina College of Pharmacy, Medical University of
    South Carolina Campus
Clinical Pharmacy Specialist, Pediatrics
Medical University of South Carolina Children's Hospital
Charleston, South Carolina

Annie M. Rakoczy, PharmD
Director of Clinical Pharmacy
PGY1 Residency Coordinator, Managed Care
HealthSpring
Nashville, Tennessee

Jo Ellen Rodgers, PharmD, FCCP, BCPS (AQ Cardiology)
Clinical Associate Professor
PGY2 Residency Program Director, Cardiology
Clinical Specialist, Cardiology
University of North Carolina Eshelman School of Pharmacy
Chapel Hill, North Carolina

Philip T. Rodgers, PharmD, FCCP, BCPS, CPP
Clinical Associate Professor
University of North Carolina Eshelman School of Pharmacy
PGY2 Residency Program Director, Ambulatory Care
Duke University Hospital
Director of Pharmacy Education
North Carolina Duke Area Health Education Center
Durham, North Carolina

Mollie A. Scott, PharmD, BCPS, CPP
Director of Professional Education and Clinical Associate Professor
University of North Carolina Eshelman School of Pharmacy–Asheville
    Campus
University of North Carolina School of Medicine
Asheville, North Carolina

Kelly M. Smith, PharmD, BCPS, FASHP, FCCP
Associate Dean, Academic and Student Affairs
Associate Professor, Pharmacy Practice and Science
Director, Residency Program Advancement
University of Kentucky College of Pharmacy
Lexington, Kentucky

David W. Stewart, PharmD, BCPS
Assistant Professor
PGY2 Residency Program Director, Internal Medicine
Clinical Specialist, Internal Medicine
Bill Gatton College of Pharmacy, East Tennessee State University
Johnson City, Tennessee

Michael C. Thomas, PharmD, BCPS
Assistant Professor
South University School of Pharmacy–Savannah Campus
Clinical Specialist, Emergency Medicine
St. Joseph's/Candler Health System
Savannah, Georgia

Jeffrey M. Tingen, PharmD, MBA, BCPS
Clinical Assistant Professor
University of Michigan College of Pharmacy
Ann Arbor, Michigan

Anna M. Wodlinger Jackson, PharmD, BCPS (AQ Cardiology)
PGY1 Residency Program Director
Clinical Pharmacy Specialist
Inova Fairfax Hospital
Falls Church, Virginia

REVIEWERS

David G. Bowyer, RPh
Director of Experiential Education
University of Charleston School of Pharmacy
Charleston, West Virginia

Susan P. Bruce, PharmD, BCPS
Chair and Associate Professor, Pharmacy Practice
Northeastern Ohio Universities Colleges of Medicine and Pharmacy
Rootstown, Ohio

Valerie A. Coppenrath, PharmD, BCPS
Assistant Professor of Pharmacy Practice
Massachusetts College of Pharmacy and Health Sciences–Worcester
Worcester, Massachusetts

Mitchell R. Emerson, PhD
Associate Dean of Academic Programs
Midwestern University College of Pharmacy–Glendale
Glendale, Arizona

Kari Furtek, PharmD, BCPS, AAHIVE
Clinical Assistant Professor
Northeastern University–School of Pharmacy
Boston, Massachusetts

Evan R. Horton, PharmD
Assistant Professor of Pharmacy Practice
Massachusetts College of Pharmacy and Health Sciences–Worcester
Worcester, Massachusetts

Sarah A. Parnapy Jawaid, PharmD
Associate Professor of Pharmacy Practice
Shenandoah University Bernard J. Dunn School of Pharmacy
Winchester, Virginia

Mark S. Johnson, PharmD, BCPS
Associate Professor and Director of Postgraduate Education
Shenandoah University Bernard J. Dunn School of Pharmacy
Winchester, Virginia

Harold L. Kirschenbaum, MS, PharmD
Associate Dean for Professional Affairs; Professor of Pharmacy Practice
Long Island University Arnold and Marie Schwartz College of Pharmacy
    and Health Sciences
Brooklyn, New York

Jason W. Lancaster, PharmD, BCPS
Assistant Clinical Professor
Northeastern University School of Pharmacy
Boston, Massachusetts

Stefanie C. Nigro, PharmD, C-TTS
Assistant Clinical Professor
University of Connecticut School of Pharmacy
Storrs, Connecticut

Nga T. Pham, PharmD
Assistant Clinical Professor of Pharmacy Practice
Northeastern University School of Pharmacy
Boston, Massachusetts

Jennifer L. Robertson, PharmD
Clinical Assistant Professor
Elizabeth City State University and UNC Eshelman School of Pharmacy
Elizabeth City, North Carolina

Rebekah E. Sherman, PharmD, CDE
Assistant Clinical Professor
Northeastern University School of Pharmacy
Boston, Massachusetts

Sarah A. Spinler, PharmD, BCPS (AQ Cardiology)
Residency Programs Director
Philadelphia College of Pharmacy
Philadelphia, Pennsylvania

Maria A. Summa, PharmD, RPh, BPCS
Associate Professor of Pharmacy Practice and Administration
Saint Joseph College, School of Pharmacy
Hartford, Connecticut

Trent G. Towne, PharmD, BCPS
Assistant Professor of Clinical Pharmacy and Residency Program Director
Philadelphia College of Pharmacy
Philadelphia, Pennsylvania

The Case for Pharmacy Residencies

L. Brian Cross, Section Editor

CHAPTER 1

Introduction to Postgraduate Training Opportunities

Michael A. Crouch

You can always amend a big plan, but you can never expand a little one.

—**Harry Truman**

QUESTIONS TO PONDER

1. Why should someone consider postgraduate training?
2. What is the primary purpose of a pharmacy residency?
3. How do pharmacy residencies and fellowships differ?
4. Who should consider an additional degree?

The term *postgraduate training* in pharmacy describes additional preparation that one completes after a doctor of pharmacy (PharmD) degree. Combined degree programs—for example, merging a PharmD with master of public health (MPH) or doctor of philosophy (PhD)—achieve the same goals as certain postgraduate training but do so in a way that allows individuals to complete two programs concurrently over a shorter period. After graduation, a variety of postgraduate training opportunities exist, including additional degrees, fellowships, and residencies. Certificate programs (e.g., immunizations) also fall under the heading of postgraduate training, although they are limited in scope. The purpose of this chapter is to provide a brief overview of major types of postgraduate training, examine reasons to consider additional experience, and characterize how pharmacy residencies differ from other postgraduate opportunities. Subsequent chapters in Section I provide details regarding the various pharmacy residencies available to graduates.

REASONS TO CONSIDER POSTGRADUATE TRAINING

The motivation to pursue postgraduate training varies depending on the student's areas of interest. Irrespective of the chosen career path, the rationale to complete additional training revolves around a sincere desire to excel as a clinician, researcher, and/or pharmacy leader. Residency training in general prepares individuals to be a pharmacy practice leader, although some advocate the combination of a residency/master of science (MS) to prepare one uniquely for leadership roles.[1] The PharmD/master of business administration (MBA) can also serve this purpose in certain situations.

A student pharmacist should consider a pharmacy residency to expand his or her clinical skills.

A student pharmacist should consider a pharmacy residency to expand his or her clinical skills. For those who have not yet chosen an area of practice, postgraduate training can help to explore the various fields of pharmacy practice and potential career opportunities. Additionally, individuals who complete a residency program are more competitive for clinical positions that provide direct patient care. Residency training is becoming a standard that is necessary for pharmacists to provide high-quality direct patient care. For more discussion on the benefits of residency training, see Chapter 2, "The Value of Residency Training and Vision for the Future."

For individuals interested in becoming a clinical pharmacy scientist, an additional degree (e.g., PhD, MS, MPH), fellowship, or both is necessary to develop requisite research skills. These programs differ based on the number of training years, thesis/dissertation requirements, and funding to support the program.[2]

RESIDENCIES

A pharmacy residency is an organized postgraduate training program in a distinct area of pharmacy practice.[2] Residencies can take place in several healthcare environments, including the hospital, community pharmacy, long-term care facility, ambulatory care clinic, and managed care organization, among others. Some programs may be associated with or contained within a college or school of pharmacy. School-based residency programs may have greater emphasis on teaching and/or develop residents into academicians.

A pharmacy residency serves as a bridge between pharmacy school and proficient clinical practice.

The primary goal of a pharmacy residency is to develop direct patient care skills. As compared to fellowships (discussed later in this chapter), approximately 80% of time in a residency is devoted to clinical practice. A pharmacy residency serves as

Table 1-1 Notable Dates in the Development of Pharmacy Residencies

1930s	Internships
1948	ASHP* standards for internships developed
1962	ASHP accreditation standards for hospital pharmacy residencies adopted
1992	ASHP commissions a project that led to the Residency Learning System (RLS)
2005	New accreditation standards regarding postgraduate year one (PGY1) and postgraduate year two (PGY2) residencies (enacted in 2007)

*ASHP: American Society of Health-System Pharmacists
Source: Adapted from American Society of Health-System Pharmacists. History of residency training. http://www.ashp.org/menu/Residents/GeneralInfo/ResidencyHistory.aspx. Accessed March 31, 2011.

a bridge between pharmacy school and proficient clinical practice. **Table 1-1** outlines important dates in the development of pharmacy residencies.[3]

The initial purpose of pharmacy residencies was to train hospital pharmacy leaders and managers. In subsequent years, beginning in the late 1960s, the aim of residencies changed, with the primary purpose being to develop clinical pharmacists. Starting in the 1970s and continuing into the 1980s, accreditation standards were developed.[4] More recently, the American Society of Health-System Pharmacists (ASHP) House of Delegates and the American College of Clinical Pharmacy (ACCP) adopted the stance that by the year 2020 the completion of an ASHP-accredited residency should be a requirement for all new college of pharmacy graduates who will be providing direct patient care.[5,6] The major barrier to reach this goal is an insufficient number of residency positions to meet student demand. To help meet this shortcoming, a change in the residency practice model has been proposed that includes a higher resident-to-preceptor ratio and different service roles for residents.[7]

ASHP accredits residency programs, although there remain a fair number of programs that choose not to go through this accreditation process. ASHP released new accreditation standards in the fall of 2005, which took effect in 2007.[8] One of the most pronounced changes within these standards was the establishment and differentiation of postgraduate year one (PGY1) and postgraduate year two (PGY2) residencies. Pharmacy graduates seeking an accredited pharmacy residency can consider PGY1 residencies only, specifically those occurring in the institutional, community pharmacy, or managed care areas. **Figure 1-1** compares PGY1 and PGY2 residencies in regards to depth of knowledge, skills, abilities, and patient–practice focus. Subsequent chapters in this section of the book provide details regarding these residency programs. Accredited residencies have a higher perceived value since

Pharmacy graduates seeking an accredited pharmacy residency can consider PGY1 residencies only, specifically those occurring in the institutional, community pharmacy, or managed care areas.

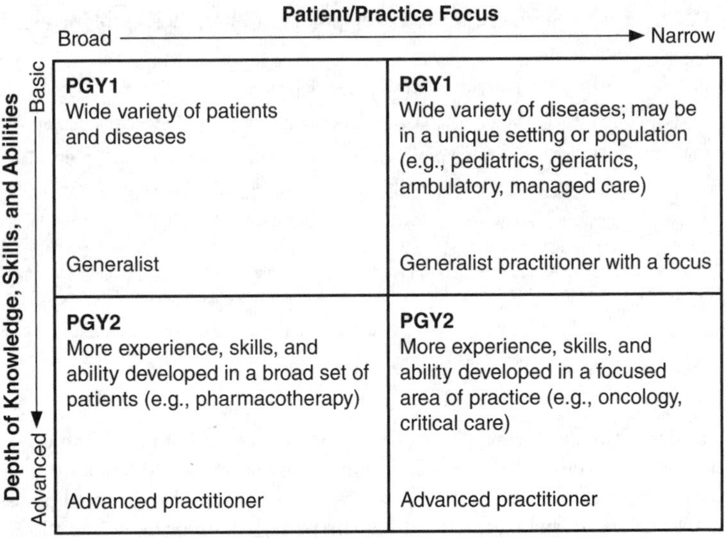

Patient/Practice Focus

Broad ——————————————————————————————→ Narrow

	PGY1	PGY1
Basic	Wide variety of patients and diseases	Wide variety of diseases; may be in a unique setting or population (e.g., pediatrics, geriatrics, ambulatory, managed care)
	Generalist	Generalist practitioner with a focus
	PGY2	PGY2
	More experience, skills, and ability developed in a broad set of patients (e.g., pharmacotherapy)	More experience, skills, and ability developed in a focused area of practice (e.g., oncology, critical care)
Advanced	Advanced practitioner	Advanced practitioner

Figure 1-1: Current Pharmacy Residency Model

Source: Teeters JL. New ASHP pharmacy residency accreditation standards. *Am J Health Syst Pharm.* 2006;63:1012–1018. © 2006, American Society of Health-System Pharmacists, Inc. All rights reserved. Reprinted with permission. (R1034)

they help to ensure a minimal standard of quality. Importantly, individuals must complete an accredited PGY1 residency to be eligible for a PGY2 program. Based on the most recent accreditation standards, both PGY1 and PGY2 ASHP-accredited programs now go through a standardized process to match applicants with pharmacy residency programs, which is discussed in Chapter 16, "The Residency Matching Program."

OTHER POSTGRADUATE TRAINING OPPORTUNITIES

For individuals interested in postgraduate training, there are various options other than pharmacy residencies to consider. These opportunities, listed in the following pages, prepare graduates for expanded research and/or business skills. **Figure 1-2** provides an overview of contemporary training programs that prepare one to be a clinical pharmacy scientist.

• Fellowships

A fellowship is a directed, highly individualized postgraduate training program that is usually research based and less clinically oriented than a residency program. Fellowships may occur in a variety of settings, including colleges or schools of pharmacy and the pharmaceutical industry. A research

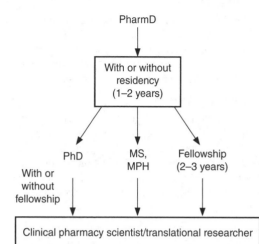

Figure 1-2: Contemporary Approaches to Become a Clinical Pharmacy Scientist

PharmD: doctor of pharmacy; PhD: doctor of philosophy; MS: master of science; MPH: master of public health

Source: Modified from Fagan SC, Touchette D, Smith JA, et al. The state of science and research in clinical pharmacy. *Pharmacotherapy*. 2006;26:1027–1040. Reprinted with permission.

fellowship is designed to prepare the participant to function as an independent investigator.[1] In these types of programs, research accounts for approximately 80% of the fellow's time. Importantly, there are an increasing number of nonresearch fellowships available in the pharmaceutical industry. In general, fellowships take a minimum of two years to complete.

> Research accounts for approximately 80% of the fellow's time.

• Doctor of Philosophy

A doctor of philosophy (PhD) is the highest academic degree an individual can earn. A PhD candidate may complete the advanced degree concurrently with a PharmD or upon graduation. The primary purpose of a PhD is to prepare graduates for professional roles in research. It consists of course work followed by focused, substantial research culminating in a formal, published dissertation.[1] A PhD generally takes four to six years to complete, but it may be shorter if completed concurrently with a PharmD.

• Master of Science

A master of science (MS) may be completed after or simultaneous with a PharmD. This degree consists of formal course work that may include biostatistics, clinical trial design, and other relevant discipline-specific topics.[1] This represents another option to develop research skills. The usual amount of time needed to complete an MS, if not accomplished concurrently with a PharmD, is two years. A formal, written thesis may be required.

• Master of Public Health

A master of public health (MPH) focuses on public health practice, and candidates may complete it in tandem or after the PharmD. If it is completed concurrently, it may require only one additional year of study. Similar to the PhD and MS, the MPH includes required course work. In addition to enhancing research skills, a traditional MPH allows candidates to focus in one of six core areas, including biostatistics, epidemiology, health service administration, health education, behavioral science, and environmental science.[1,9] If the Council on Education for Public Health (CEPH; www.ceph .org) accredits the program, there is thesis and practicum requirements.[9]

• Master of Business Administration

The master of business administration (MBA) degree is suited for students interested in the management of human or other business resources. If completed concurrently with a PharmD, it may require only one additional year of study. Conversely, MBA degrees completed after graduation are full-time (two years), accelerated, part-time, or executive programs (e.g., weekends). Specialized areas of MBA programs include accounting, economics, finance, and management, among others.

KEY POINTS

- Postgraduate training allows one to develop expertise as a clinician, researcher, and/or leader.

- The primary goal of a pharmacy residency is to develop clinical skills; it serves as a bridge between pharmacy school and proficient clinical practice.

- A research fellowship is designed to prepare the participant to function as an independent investigator; there are an increasing number of nonresearch fellowships available in the pharmaceutical industry.

- Additional or combined degree programs help one develop research or business skills.

REFERENCES

1. Hunt ML. Aspiring leaders should consider M.S.-residency programs. *Am J Health Syst Pharm*. 2000;57:2169.
2. Fagan SC, Touchette D, Smith JA, et al. The state of science and research in clinical pharmacy. *Pharmacotherapy*. 2006;26:1027–1040.
3. American Society of Health-System Pharmacists. History of residency training. http://www.ashp.org/menu/Residents/GeneralInfo/ResidencyHistory.aspx. Accessed March 31, 2011.
4. Ray MD. Pharmacy residency training: proposal for a fourth wave. *Am J Health Syst Pharm*.1997;54:2116–2121.
5. Murphy JE, Nappi JM, Bosso JA, et al. American College of Clinical Pharmacy's vision of the future: postgraduate pharmacy residency training as a prerequisite for direct patient care practice. *Pharmacotherapy*. 2006;26:722–733.
6. American Society of Health-System Pharmacists. Professional policies approved by the 2007 ASHP House of Delegates. *Am J Health Syst Pharm*. 2007;64:e68–e71.
7. Ashby DM, McMahon PO. Need for changes in the residency practice module. *Am J Health Syst Pharm*. 2011;68:19.
8. Teeters JL. New ASHP pharmacy residency accreditation standards. *Am J Health Syst Pharm*. 2006;63:1012–1018.
9. Council on Education for Public Health. Accreditation criteria. http://www.ceph .org/pg_accreditation_criteria.htm. Accessed March 31, 2011.

CHAPTER 2

The Value of Residency Training and Vision for the Future

Michael C. Thomas

Education is learning what you didn't even know you didn't know.

—Daniel J. Boorstin

QUESTIONS TO PONDER

1. How are pharmacy residencies different from advanced pharmacy practice experiences?
2. Why is experience necessary to become a proficient clinical practitioner?
3. Who benefits from residency training?
4. What are the rewards of a residency program?
5. Is residency training consistent with the vision of pharmacy organizations?

EDUCATION WITHOUT APPLICATION IS A WASTE

Pharmacy education and the pharmacy profession continue to change to meet the needs of the healthcare system. Most recently, the PharmD was decided upon as the required education path for aspiring pharmacists entering pharmacy school in the 2000 to 2001 school year.[1] Pharmacy schools bear the responsibility of graduating practitioners with the competency to ensure optimal patient safety and medication use outcomes in any setting.[1] Indeed, this is a tall order, and great effort is placed in professional curricula to expose students to a vast amount of information. Students begin to realize complete application of this information during advanced pharmacy practice experiences (APPEs), but the initial application may begin as early as the introductory pharmacy practice experiences (IPPEs) in the community and institutional settings. During these experiences, students begin to apply what they have learned to advance the care of patients. The rotations are designed to provide exposure to different types of pharmacy practice. By graduation, therefore, students have been exposed to a great volume of didactic knowledge that has been only partly applied in patient care activities. Examinations are necessary assessment tools in the classroom setting; however, there is not an immediate effect on patient care, and they may not be a true test of application even when simulated. Pharmacy practice experiences require that students apply their knowledge daily, making these experiences the most important assessment tool.

Application of knowledge incorporates attitudes, therapeutic knowledge, problem solving, and social skills to ensure optimal patient care. At best, students are novices at pulling all of these pieces together, not because of lack of knowledge, but because of lack of experience. The application of knowledge in everyday situations provides meaning and perspective to the knowledge students have gained in the classroom. Both knowledge and patient care experiences are required to hone clinical skills. Many recent graduates may not believe pharmacy school has prepared them to provide direct patient care independently with confidence. The number one factor influencing students to pursue a pharmacy residency is a desire to gain knowledge and experience.[2]

> **The number one factor influencing students to pursue a pharmacy residency is a desire to gain knowledge and experience.**

Acquiring clinical skills for physicians has been described as "see one, do one, and teach one."[3] Though a simplified view, at its core are lessons that can be learned if we change "one" to "many." Introductory and advanced pharmacy practice experiences provide students with the opportunity to see a variety of pharmacists, settings, patient populations, and disease types. This exposure will allow students to identify knowledge gaps or opportunities to deepen understanding, even when the experiences may be more observation than action.

The second most cited reason for pursuing a residency is to build confidence.[2] One way to build confidence is by taking care of many patients through direct patient care. Residency experiences allow for the practice of pharmacy with appropriate mentoring and assessment that expand the learners' clinical repertoire. A residency also allows one to discern when clinical situations are beyond the expertise of the resident.[4] An effective preceptor can model clinical skills and provide valuable teaching opportunities for the resident. Pharmacists who have completed a residency have provided direct patient care to many individuals. They have moved from

> **The second most cited reason for pursuing a residency is to build confidence.**

"see many" to "do many" in their postgraduate year one (PGY1) residency and are prepared to provide direct patient care independently or to pursue specialized training via a postgraduate year two (PGY2) residency or fellowship (see Chapter 7, "Postgraduate Year Two (PGY2) Residency Programs," for further discussion). This stage does not stop with residency training, but it continues throughout one's professional career. Through residency training, these pharmacists have gained the experience necessary to provide direct patient care. They are able to incorporate new knowledge into the provision of optimal patient care to future patients.

Pharmacists, by the nature of the profession, are teachers. They teach patients, caregivers, healthcare professionals at all levels, students, residents, and other pharmacists. Oftentimes, residents have their first teaching opportunities during postgraduate training programs. They may help precept student pharmacists completing IPPEs or APPEs, or provide more structured education in a classroom setting. Some residency programs also provide teaching certificate programs, which allow for the development of effective teaching and learning strategies.[5] They may teach students participating in introductory or advanced practice experiences, provide didactic lectures, deliver continuing education programs, or offer community service activities to the public (e.g., health screenings and brown bag events). Teaching is a skill that must be practiced to be effective. Residency training affords opportunities to begin learning and practicing teaching techniques in a variety of settings.

NO SUBSTITUTE FOR EXPERIENCE

A clinical pharmacist's proficiency in the practice of pharmacy requires formal training and experience beyond pharmacy school.[4] PGY1 residency programs accredited by the American Society of Health-System Pharmacists (ASHP) requires residents to take an active role in the medication use process by providing optimal pharmaceutical care; developing leadership and management skills; educating patients, healthcare professionals, and student pharmacists; and effectively using information technology in the care of patients.[6] The resident is clearly expected to take an active role in patient care and serve essential functions within the institution. When these outcomes are realized, the resident has gained a unique set of skills through the rigor and structure of a residency program. Residents learn the organizational structure and flow of the healthcare system and discover the impact pharmacists make on patient care within the institution. Concepts and procedures that were foreign before residency training become clear as residents practice pharmacy and grow as professionals. These foundational concepts and skills become part of the fabric of the practitioner's expertise and serve as a point of reference for future challenges.

Residents are expected to provide optimal pharmaceutical care. The first step in this process is accomplished by taking responsibility for patient care. This responsibility becomes a driving force for learning. To attain a high level of patient care proficiency, direction must be given by someone more

To attain a high level of patient care proficiency, direction must be given by someone more experienced.

experienced.[3] Structured residency programs provide opportunities to practice pharmacy within a network of skilled preceptors. Effective precepting guides learning and proficiency in the care of patients and allows the resident to model the preceptor's effective clinical skills.

During the minimum 12-month experience as a resident, there may be opportunities to appreciate aspects of the healthcare system beyond traditional pharmacy services. The general atmosphere supports learning. This is a time when the budding professional can appreciate the contribution of other healthcare professionals to the care of patients. The resident can experience firsthand the medication use process and see how patients are ultimately affected at the bedside. There may be opportunities to observe surgeries, diagnostic or interventional procedures, therapeutic techniques, and general patient care. These experiences add to residents' understanding of the complete care of patients and how medications fit into this paradigm of patient care.

BENEFIT IS MORE THAN RESIDENT DEEP

Graduates of a pharmacy residency program reap numerous benefits as they gain experience in direct patient care, education, and leadership, and as they develop an understanding of how the healthcare system functions. Employers desire or, in some cases, require residency-trained clinical pharmacists for entry-level positions. If the resident wants to pursue a specialized focus and complete a PGY2, the completion of a PGY1 is a prerequisite. Residency training includes experiences that take years to attain outside of a structured program, if they are attained at all. Beyond value to the resident, there are also benefits to patients, the profession of pharmacy, and the host institution. These benefits are detailed in the American College of Clinical Pharmacy (ACCP) white paper dedicated to this topic.[5]

The direct benefit to the institution that hosts a residency program is expanded staffing capacity. The program allows added flexibility and capacity for the operations manager to schedule personnel within the pharmacy or the hospital to support clinical endeavors. Residents may also aid in the expansion of clinical services by piloting new services or by extending existing services. Other benefits are related to direct or indirect revenue generation. Examples of direct revenues are financial support from higher education institutions to train doctor of pharmacy students during pharmacy practice experiences, Medicare pass-through funds for training residents, and the generation of billable services (e.g., clinical trial recruitment, contractual work). Indirect revenue is realized with reduced training costs if residents continue employment at their place of residency and improved pay-for-performance benchmarks because of clinical interventions made by residents. Residents may also contribute by conducting medication use evaluations, research projects, and by developing policies, procedures, or standardized order sets.

Patients also benefit from residency programs. Patients equate encountering trained professionals with increased capacity to deliver excellent care. Patients also benefit directly because of an institution's increased capacity to provide pharmacy services, either directly or indirectly by residents. Patients benefit when interventions and recommendations made by residents improve their care.[5] Residents may also participate in community service activities, such as health fairs or brown bag events, which are highly visible benefits to patients.

Residency programs also benefit the profession as a whole. Residency graduates have the skills and expertise that enable them to provide direct patient care, measure and demonstrate important research metrics, and work within an interdisciplinary team in complex environments. All of these benefits are consistent with the vision that having a pharmacist license will not be sufficient to hospital and health-system pharmacy practice in the future.[6,7]

> By the year 2020, all entry-level positions with direct patient care responsibilities may require residency training.

VISION FOR THE FUTURE

Both the ACCP and the ASHP have published long-term visions for pharmacy practice.[6,7] By the year 2020, all entry-level positions with direct patient care responsibilities may require residency training.[7,8]

• American College of Clinical Pharmacy's Vision

The ACCP Task Force on Residencies cites a number of reasons for requiring residency training for all pharmacists who provide direct patient care.[7] Pharmacy school graduates may not have sufficient ability to manage complex drug therapy. Additionally, payers and regulatory bodies may require advanced training for privileging and payment (similar to the medical model). Lastly, direct patient care provided by pharmacists is anticipated to become the standard of care by 2020. Benefits of completing a residency include clinical skill development, expanded marketability as an employee, diverse practice experiences, networking, an increased role of pharmacists in new and emerging areas, and educational opportunities. In addition, pharmacists with postgraduate training are more involved in their profession, submitting scholarly contributions, assuming leadership roles within pharmacy organizations, and becoming lifelong learners. The ACCP task force believes that residency training is the most efficient mechanism to move student pharmacists from merely competent to highly proficient practitioners.

• American Society of Health-System Pharmacists' Vision

The ASHP House of Delegates passed a resolution to support the position to require pharmacy residency training by the year 2020.[8] In its vision for the pharmacy work force, licensure alone will no longer be sufficient to practice in the hospital or health-system setting.[6] Residencies are intense, practice-based training opportunities. Clinical skills are developed through mentoring and holding the resident accountable, so that he or she is better prepared to accept an entry-level position. The enriched experiences that develop expertise in graduates of pharmacy residency programs empower them to provide direct patient care in a complex interdisciplinary environment and to demonstrate their effectiveness using relevant objectives.

KEY POINTS

• The role of the pharmacist is clearly changing within the complex healthcare system, and pharmacy school graduates need advanced training to provide efficient direct patient care.

• Experience is a cornerstone to the development of a practitioner and, when guided by a knowledgeable preceptor during residency training, the resident's value and growth will be optimized.

• Residency training benefits residents, patients, the institution hosting the residency program, and the profession of pharmacy.

• The ultimate benefits of residency training include a better-prepared clinical work force able to meet the challenges within the complex healthcare system.

• Major pharmacy organizations have called for residency training to be a minimum standard for direct patient care by the year 2020.

REFERENCES

1. Accreditation Council for Pharmacy Education. Accreditation standards and guidelines for the professional program in pharmacy leading to the doctor of pharmacy degree. http://www.acpe-accredit.org/pdf/finals2007guidelines2.0.pdf. Accessed March 31, 2011.
2. Fit KE, Padiyara RS, Rabi SM, Burkiewicz JS. Factors influencing pursuit of residency training. *Am J Health Syst Pharm*. 2005;62:2226–2235.
3. Cooke M, Irby DM, Sullivan W, Ludmerer KM. American medical education 100 years after the Flexner report. *N Engl J Med*. 2006;355:1339–1344.
4. Burke JM, Miller WA, Spencer AP, et al. Clinical pharmacist competencies. *Pharmacotherapy*. 2008;28:806–815.
5. Smith KM, Sorensen T, Connor KA, et al. Value of conducting pharmacy residency training—the organizational perspective. http://www.accp.com/docs/positions/whitePapers/Pharm3012e_ACCP-ResTraining.pdf. Accessed March 31, 2011.
6. American Society of Health-System Pharmacists. ASHP long-range vision for the pharmacy work force in hospitals and health systems: ensuring the best use of medicines in hospitals and health systems. *Am J Health Syst Pharm*. 2007;64:1320–1330.
7. Murphy JE, Nappi JM, Bosso JA, et al. American College of Clinical Pharmacy's vision of the future: postgraduate pharmacy residency training as a prerequisite for direct patient care practice. *Pharmacotherapy*. 2006;26:722–733.
8. American Society of Health-System Pharmacists. Professional policies approved by the 2007 ASHP House of Delegates. *Am J Health Syst Pharm*. 2007;64:e68–e71.

CHAPTER 3

Postgraduate Year One (PGY1) Pharmacy Residency Programs

Dominic P. Ragucci

Experience: that most brutal of teachers. But you learn, my God do you learn.

—C.S. Lewis

QUESTIONS TO PONDER

1. What is the history behind pharmacy residency programs in the hospital/health-system setting?

2. Why should one consider a pharmacy residency program in the hospital/health-system setting over other types of first-year residency opportunities?

3. What are some unique learning opportunities available to pharmacy residents in the hospital/health-system setting?

4. What factors should be considered when comparing different postgraduate year one (PGY1) pharmacy residencies in the hospital/health-system setting?

Hospital/health-system pharmacy residencies have a long history, dating back to the 1930s with the internship at the University of Michigan in Ann Arbor under the supervision of Harvey A.K. Whitney and Edward C. Watts.[1] The focus, terminology, and accreditation standards for residency training have evolved over time (see Chapter 1, "Introduction to Postgraduate Training Opportunities"). The greater emphasis on direct patient care activities began in the 1970s leading to the first American Society of Health-System Pharmacists (ASHP, known as the American Society of Hospital Pharmacists at the time) Accreditation Standards for Residency Training in Clinical Pharmacy in 1980. In 1992, the pharmacy practice residency became the standard training experience emphasizing pharmaceutical care. Today, *postgraduate year one* (PGY1) and *postgraduate year two* (PGY2) is accepted terminology to clarify the concepts of generalists and advanced practitioners. The PGY1 pharmacy residency is designed to provide a general pharmacy experience for pharmacy school graduates, as compared to the PGY2 pharmacy residency that provides specialized or advanced training after a PGY1 residency. ASHP recently released standards related to PGY1 international accreditation.[2]

The PGY1 pharmacy residency further develops clinical skills fostered during students' advanced pharmacy practice experiences. Upon completion of the PGY1 pharmacy residency, residents should be well prepared for generalist positions as well as additional PGY2 pharmacy residency training. Hospital/health-system accredited PGY1 pharmacy residency programs provide an ideal environment to accomplish the six required outcomes published in the Residency Learning System (RLS) that are required for successful completion of the PGY1 experience (**Table 3-1**).[3] Chapter 4,

---

Table 3-1 Educational Outcomes for PGY1 Pharmacy Residency Programs

Required Outcomes

Outcome R1:	Manage and improve the medication-use process.
Outcome R2:	Provide evidence-based, patient-centered medication therapy management with interdisciplinary teams.
Outcome R3:	Exercise leadership and practice management skills.
Outcome R4:	Demonstrate project management skills.
Outcome R5:	Provide medication and practice-related education and training.
Outcome R6:	Utilize medical informatics.

Elective Outcomes

Outcome E1:	Conduct pharmacy practice research.
Outcome E2:	Exercise added leadership and practice management skills.
Outcome E3:	Demonstrate knowledge and skills particular to generalist practice in the home care practice environment.
Outcome E4:	Demonstrate knowledge and skills particular to generalist practice in the managed care practice environment.
Outcome E5:	Participate in the management of medical emergencies.
Outcome E6:	Provide drug information to healthcare professionals and/or the public.
Outcome E7:	Demonstrate additional competencies that contribute to working successfully in the healthcare environment.

Source: Modified from American Society of Health-System Pharmacists. Required and elective outcomes, goals, objectives, and instructional objectives for postgraduate year one (PGY1) pharmacy residency programs, 2nd edition—effective July 2008. http://www.ashp.org/DocLibrary/Accreditation/PGY1-Goals-Objectives.aspx. Accessed March 31, 2011. Reprinted with permission.

"Postgraduate Year One (PGY1) Community Pharmacy Residency Programs," and Chapter 5, "Postgraduate Year One (PGY1) Managed Care Pharmacy Residency Programs," provide detailed comparisons of outcomes between hospital/health-system-based and other PGY1 pharmacy residencies.

PGY1 outcomes are achieved with required educational goals and objectives. Individual programs may select additional elective outcomes with associated educational goals and objectives, as well (see Table 3-1). The type of hospital/health-system (e.g., teaching versus community) and the institution's available resources help shape the learning experiences to meet required and elective outcomes for individual PGY1 programs.

CONSIDERATIONS FOR PGY1 HOSPITAL/HEALTH-SYSTEM PHARMACY RESIDENCY PROGRAMS

In 2001, ASHP introduced the 2015 Initiative, which focuses on measurable goals and objectives to improve pharmacy practice in the healthcare setting by the year 2015.[4] Many of these goals and objectives directly influence the daily activities and responsibilities of pharmacists in the hospital/health-system setting. A hospital/health-system residency prepares graduates to meet ASHP's 2015 Initiative goals by further developing critical-thinking skills, interdisciplinary communication skills, and drug and disease state knowledge (**Table 3-2**).

> A hospital/health-system residency prepares graduates to meet ASHP's 2015 Initiative goals.

A pharmacy practice residency in the hospital/health-system setting provides varied and diverse experiences for new graduates who have not

Table 3-2 Goals for ASHP's 2015 Initiative	
Goal 1	Increase the extent to which pharmacists help individual hospital inpatients achieve the best use of medications.
Goal 2	Increase the extent to which health-system pharmacists help individual nonhospitalized patients achieve the best use of medications.
Goal 3	Increase the extent to which health-system pharmacists actively apply evidence-based methods to the improvement of medication therapy.
Goal 4	Increase the extent to which pharmacy departments in health systems have a significant role in improving the safety of medication use.
Goal 5	Increase the extent to which health systems apply technology effectively to improve the safety of medication use.
Goal 6	Increase the extent to which pharmacy departments in health systems engage in public health initiatives on behalf of their communities.

Source: Modified from American Society of Health-System Pharmacists. 2015 ASHP health-system pharmacy initiative. http://www.ashp.org/s_ashp/docs/files/2015_Goals_Objectives_0508.pdf. Accessed March 31, 2011. Reprinted with permission.

yet identified a practice area of interest. New graduates can continue structured training with direct supervision in multiple practice settings. Most residencies have rotations ranging from intensive to ambulatory care. Pharmacy services are provided for patients of differing acuity and complexity, exposing trainees to many different disease states and drug therapies. No more than a third of the year should be committed to one particular specialty area, ensuring a well-rounded learning experience.[3] The design of each hospital/health-system residency will vary depending on the strengths and diversity of the supporting institution.

UNIQUE ASPECTS OF PGY1 HOSPITAL/HEALTH-SYSTEM PHARMACY RESIDENCY PROGRAMS

A hospital/health-system experience offers a unique learning opportunity for residency training. A resident in this setting will have the opportunity to acquire firsthand experience participating in the medical management of acutely ill patients. Critically ill and acutely ill patients require a high level of care that is attainable only in the hospital/health-system setting. Depending on the patient mix in a specific hospital or health-system, PGY1 residents will encounter a wide range of acute and ambulatory care populations presenting with a variety of diseases and severities.

PGY1 residents will encounter a wide range of acute and ambulatory care populations.

ASHP annually recognizes practitioners who "have successfully implemented innovative systems that improve the quality of patient care and demonstrate best practices in health-system pharmacy."[5] These program initiatives enhance the hospital/health-system-based residency learning experience and encourage future innovation by those individuals exposed to best practices.

A major non rotation experience of a hospital/health-system residency includes the operational pharmacy component. Residents are expected to function as a direct care or clinical pharmacist within the pharmacy department and to staff the distribution process established at each institution. A better understanding of the distributive model enables the residents to make clinical practice decisions that best address patient care needs while considering practical implications for drug dosing, preparation, and delivery. The staffing time commitment varies among institutions based on departmental needs and established practice models.

Many programs provide pharmacy on-call services to support pharmacy personnel and other healthcare professionals for the provision of patient care. Coverage expectations for residents completing on-call duties may range from 24-hour clinical in-house coverage to weekly 24-hour, 7-days-a-week coverage with availability by pager overnight. On-call clinical activities may include emergency care/code participation, pharmacokinetic and antibiotic surveillance, targeted patient counseling, drug information services, parenteral and enteral nutrition support, and other high-alert medication monitoring. Residents receive backup support while on call with either a PGY2 pharmacy resident or a clinical pharmacist.

DIFFERENCES AMONG PGY1 HOSPITAL/HEALTH-SYSTEM PHARMACY RESIDENCY PROGRAMS

To meet the increasing demand for residency training, many new hospital/health-system residency positions have been established in settings other than academic medical centers or large health-systems. Community hospitals are able to provide valuable residency experiences in compliance with ASHP PGY1 standards for accreditation.[5] Community hospitals tend to have a greater focus on general medicine patients as compared to more specialized care patients. Limited affiliations with colleges or schools of pharmacy may make teaching opportunities more challenging to obtain. The dynamics of inter-professional rounds and collaboration are exchanged for more independent patient monitoring and communication techniques. Community hospital residencies may have fewer residents and preceptors, allowing for more individualized training and learning opportunities (e.g., longitudinal experiences, additional committee participation). Even among academic medical centers, residency experiences may differ depending on the institution. As an example, some freestanding children's hospitals offer hospital/health-system PGY1 residencies. These programs may appeal to residents with a known interest in providing pharmaceutical care to children and their caregivers, although this is not a substitute for specialty training in this area obtained through a PGY2 residency.

The size of the hospital (number of patient beds) may influence the pharmacist's role in managing the medication use system. A recent survey among 1364 hospitals in the United States showed that the size of the hospital influences pharmacist models, organizational technologies, pharmacy service coverage, and even medication therapy monitoring activites.[7] Larger hospitals (e.g., more than 600 beds) reported higher percentages for implementation of technologies, such as computerized physician/provider order entry, smart infusion pumps, and electronic medical records. In addition, they reported expanded specialty service coverage (e.g., emergency services, infectious diseases, pediatrics) and medication therapy monitoring activities compared to smaller hospitals. Most hospitals (64.7%) reported implementing a patient-centered, integrated model (pharmacists had both distribution and clinical functions); however, the percentages of hospitals having a patient-centered, integrated model compared to the clinical specialist-centered model (separate distributive and clinical specialist roles) were similar (48.4% versus 45.2%, respectively) in hospitals with at least 600 beds.[7]

Additional differences among hospital or health-system residencies include the number of residents included in the program, the number and qualifications of preceptors, and the availability of specialized PGY2 programs. Programs with a larger numbers of residents may have less flexibility with certain residency requirements (e.g., rotation schedule/structure, project selection) but may offer a better support system for out-of-state matched residents and better networking opportunities. This generalization varies from one site to the next. Smaller residency programs may have lower resident-to-preceptor ratios, which may provide greater consistency in feedback. Many residency programs in larger hospitals, or those affiliated with a college or school of pharmacy, also offer specialty PGY2 residencies and more formalized teaching instruction. Programs affiliated with a college or school of pharmacy may have increased networking opportunities for those interested in academia as well as increased teaching activities. PGY1 residents in these residencies will have opportunities to rotate through more varied rotations and interact with more specialty-trained PGY2 preceptors. Residents also will have the ability to make an early commitment to a specialty PGY2 residency program at the same institution, as established by the National Matching Services.

KEY POINTS

- Pharmacy residency programs in the hospital/health-system setting have a long, distinguished history, which continues to evolve as the pharmacists' role in managing medication therapies increases.

- A hospital/health-system pharmacy residency serves as an important process for new pharmacy practitioners to increase their depth of experience so they can more effectively manage patients in this setting.

- An individual completing a residency in a hospital/health-system setting will gain firsthand experience participating in the medical management of a diverse, acute care patient population.

- Pharmacy residency programs in the hospital/health-system setting may differ from one another based on the practice setting (academic medical center versus community hospital), size of the institution, number of residents and preceptors, and opportunities for PGY2 training.

REFERENCES

1. Letendre DE, Brooks PJ, Degenhart ML. The evolution of pharmacy residency training programs and corresponding standards of accreditation. *Pharm Pract Manag Q*. 1995;15:30–43.

2. American Society of Health-System Pharmacists. ASHP international accreditation standard for postgraduate year one (PGY1) pharmacy residency programs. http://www.ashp.org/DocLibrary/Accreditation/ASDInternationalStd010410.aspx. Accessed March 31, 2011.

3. American Society of Health-System Pharmacists. ASHP accreditation standard for postgraduate year one (PGY1) pharmacy residency programs. http://www.ashp.org/DocLibrary/Accreditation/ASD-PGY1-Standard.aspx. Accessed March 31, 2011.

4. American Society of Health-System Pharmacists. 2015 ASHP health-system pharmacy initiative. http://www.ashp.org/s_ashp/docs/files/2015_Goals_Objectives_0508.pdf. Accessed March 31, 2011.

5. American Society of Health-System Pharmacists. ASHP best practices award in health-system pharmacy. http://www.ashpadvantage.com/bestpractices. Accessed March 31, 2011.

6. Paciullo CA, Moranville MP, Suffoletta TJ. Pharmacy practice residency programs in community hospitals. *Am J Health Syst Pharm.* 2010;66:536–559.

7. Pederson CA, Schneider PJ, Scheckelhoff DJ. ASHP national survey of pharmacy practice in hospital settings: monitoring and patient education—2009. *Am J Health Syst Pharm.* 2010;67:542–558.

CHAPTER 4

Postgraduate Year One (PGY1) Community Pharmacy Residency Programs

Jean-Venable "Kelly" Goode

I skate to where the puck is going to be, not to where it has been.

—Wayne Gretzky

QUESTIONS TO PONDER

1. Why should a student consider a postgraduate year one (PGY1) Community Pharmacy Residency Program?

2. What are the differences between a PGY1 Community Pharmacy Residency Program and other first-year pharmacy residencies?

3. How does an applicant choose a PGY1 Community Pharmacy Residency Program?

4. What kinds of positions are available after completion of a PGY1 Community Pharmacy Residency Program?

Residency training in community pharmacies is a new concept when compared to residency training in the institutional setting, which has existed for more than half a century. However, the importance of training future change agents for community pharmacy practice cannot be overstated. Pharmacists in community pharmacy practice have enormous potential to affect direct patient care. At a residency stakeholder roundtable discussion in 2005, the participants acknowledged "the

Pharmacists in community pharmacy practice have enormous potential to affect direct patient care.

23

huge opportunity for community pharmacists to make a positive impact on patient care due to their accessibility to the public."[1]

The Community Pharmacy Residency Program (CPRP) was established in 1986 by the American Pharmacists Association (APhA) with the following purpose: "The CPRP strives to develop creative and innovative pharmacy practice leaders who will be able to meet the challenges presented by the readily changing healthcare system, the implementation of pharmaceutical care, and the needs of society for improved monitoring of therapeutic outcomes."[2]

Originally, there were five community pharmacy residency sites, which graduated six residents in the first year of the program. In 1999, APhA entered into a partnership with the American Society of Health-System Pharmacists (ASHP) to begin accreditation of CPRPs. As of 2010, there were 71 PGY1 CPRPs (accredited and nonaccredited) with more than 100 residency training sites.[3] Practice training sites are chain, supermarket, independent, and healthcare system pharmacies. The majority of the programs are affiliated with colleges or schools of pharmacy. Additionally, a handful of established CPRPs are exploring methods for offering additional education and training related to community pharmacy practice, including PGY2 Community Pharmacy Practice Residencies, PGY2 Academic Pharmacy Practice Residencies, Community Pharmacy Practice Fellowships, and Community-Based Participatory Research Fellowships.

COMMUNITY PHARMACY RESIDENCY PROGRAM CONSIDERATIONS

> Student pharmacists should consider a community residency if they are interested in innovative direct patient care in this setting.

Student pharmacists should consider a community residency if they are interested in innovative direct patient care in this setting. APhA conducted a survey in 2000 to analyze the experiences of residents and revealed reasons for choosing a community pharmacy practice residency.[4] Since that time APhA has conducted an annual resident exit survey. The majority of residents revealed that the most important factor influencing their choice to pursue a community pharmacy residency over other types of residencies was a preference for direct patient care. Other important factors included prior community pharmacy practice experience, a sense that community practice would be worthwhile, a desire to develop innovative pharmacy services, and involvement with the many changes community pharmacy is currently undergoing. Pharmacy school graduates should choose a community pharmacy residency if they are interested in direct patient care, innovative practice, and advancing this practice setting.

UNIQUE ASPECTS OF COMMUNITY PHARMACY RESIDENCIES

Community Pharmacy Residency Programs are classified as a PGY1 residency by ASHP–APhA. PGY1 residencies are designed to build on the knowledge and skills gained from an accredited professional pharmacy degree program. Residents completing community pharmacy residencies will acquire outcome competencies that mirror the outcomes for the PGY1 Pharmacy Residency conducted in an inpatient setting. **Table 4-1**

Table 4-1 Comparison of Educational Outcomes Between PGY1 CPRPs and PGY1 Pharmacy Residency Programs

PGY1 CPRPs	*PGY1 Pharmacy Residency Programs*
Required Outcomes	
Outcome R1: Manage and improve the medication-use process.	Outcome R1: Manage and improve the medication-use process.
Outcome R2: Provide evidence-based, patient-centered care and collaborate with other healthcare professionals to optimize patient care.	Outcome R2: Provide evidence-based, patient-centered medication therapy management with interdisciplinary teams.
Outcome R3: Exercise leadership and practice management skills.	Outcome R3: Exercise leadership and practice management skills.
Outcome R4: Demonstrate project management skills.	Outcome R4: Demonstrate project management skills.
Outcome R5: Provide medication and practice-related information, education, and/or training.	Outcome R5: Provide medication and practice-related education and training.
Outcome R6: Utilize medical informatics.	Outcome R6: Utilize medical informatics.
Elective Outcomes (Matched by Content)	
Outcome E1: Provide public health programs for health improvement, wellness, and disease prevention to the community.	
Outcome E2: Participate in planning for and/or management of medical and public health emergencies.	Outcome E5: Participate in the management of medical emergencies.
Outcome E3: Conduct pharmacy practice research.	Outcome E1: Conduct pharmacy practice research.
Outcome E4: Exercise additional leadership and practice management skills.	Outcome E2: Exercise added leadership and practice management skills.

Table 4-1 Comparison of Educational Outcomes Between PGY1 CPRPs and PGY1 Pharmacy Residency Programs (*Continued*)

PGY1 CPRPs	PGY1 Pharmacy Residency Programs
Outcome E5: Demonstrate knowledge and skills for successful community practice interface with the managed care or self-insured employer environment.	Outcome E4: Demonstrate knowledge and skills particular to generalist practice in the managed care practice environment.
Outcome E6: Demonstrate skills required to function in an academic setting.	
Outcome E7: Create a community pharmacy drug information library.	
Outcome E8: Participate in the organization's formulary management processes.	
Outcome E9: Demonstrate knowledge and skills particular to generalist practice in the home care practice environment.	Outcome E3: Demonstrate knowledge and skills particular to generalist practice in the home care practice environment.
	Outcome E6: Provide drug information to healthcare professionals and/or the public.
	Outcome E7: Demonstrate additional competencies that contribute to working successfully in the healthcare environment.

Sources: Modified from American Society of Health-System Pharmacists, American Pharmacists Association. Required and elective educational outcomes, goals, objectives and instructional objectives for postgraduate year one (PGY1) community pharmacy residency programs. http://www.ashp.org/DocLibrary/Accreditation/RTPCommunityCareGoalsObj2010.aspx. Accessed March 31, 2011. Reprinted with permission; and American Society of Health-System Pharmacists. Required and elective outcomes, goals, objectives, and instructional objectives for postgraduate year one (PGY1) pharmacy residency programs, 2nd edition—effective July 2008. http://www.ashp.org/DocLibrary/Accreditation/PGY1-Goals-Objectives.aspx. Accessed March 31, 2011. Reprinted with permission.

compares the primary outcomes of a PGY1 CPRP with the PGY1 Pharmacy Residency.[5,6]

Beyond the outcomes and goals, there are some distinct differences between these residencies worth noting. A PGY1 community pharmacy residency has a structure that is longitudinal. Objectives and experiences are met over a long period of time, typically throughout the residency year. Community pharmacy practice residency programs may also offer concentrated or extended rotations for certain learning experiences, such as electives, ambulatory care clinics, or management. Another distinct difference is that community pharmacy residents receive the majority of their training and education under a primary preceptor or mentor for the entire residency program. In a community pharmacy residency, the primary preceptor or mentor is usually an established leader and innovator. The community pharmacy resident has the opportunity to work one on one with this person throughout the longitudinal learning experience.

> In a community pharmacy residency, the primary preceptor or mentor is usually an established leader and innovator.

The main distinction in the outcomes and goals between other first-year pharmacy residency programs and a PGY1 community pharmacy residency is the expectation that a community pharmacy resident learns how to develop, implement, and evaluate a new or existing patient care service in this setting. Another potential difference in the first year of a community pharmacy residency is the focus on teaching. Since colleges and schools of pharmacy administer the majority of these programs, there is usually an expectation of participation in the doctor of pharmacy curriculum.

Another difference in community residencies versus other PGY1 residencies is the availability of an informal community pharmacy practice network. Only a small number of residency programs, preceptors, and residency directors are available in the community setting, and they often are well acquainted with one another. Additionally, community pharmacy preceptors and directors are all working toward the common goal of developing innovative services and improving patient care. Entering a community pharmacy residency affords the resident the opportunity to interact and connect with the innovators and leaders in community practice settings throughout the country. Lastly, community pharmacy residency education and training enables the resident to be a practice change agent and leader. Residency graduates are prepared to meet the challenges of the rapidly changing healthcare environment.

COMMUNITY PHARMACY RESIDENCY EXPERIENCE

As noted before, accredited PGY1 Community Pharmacy Residency Programs are designed to meet the outcomes of the ASHP–APhA accreditation standard (see Table 4-1). The residency experience is conducted over a 12-month period with a minimum of 2000 hours of education and training. The program is usually designed in a longitudinal format with goals and objectives being met throughout the year. Community pharmacy residents do not necessarily have a typical week; they are always doing something different. An example of how the resident's time might be distributed is 50% in patient care, 15% in practice management, 15% in teaching, 5% in project management, 5% in professional involvement and leadership, and 10%

Table 4-2 Example Community Pharmacy Resident Responsibilities and Activities

Responsibility	Activities
Direct patient care	Medication therapy management
	Immunizations
	Screenings
	Disease management
	Patient group teaching
	Drug information
	Collaboration with other healthcare providers
Practice management	Business plan composition
	New service development and implementation
	Service marketing
	Technology use
Teaching	Student pharmacist education
	Advanced pharmacy practice experience (APPE) teaching
	Pharmacy laboratory instruction
	Pharmacist continuing education
	Health care professional education
Project management	Practice-based project development and implementation
	Poster or oral presentation
Electives	Additional patient care
	Further teaching
	Managed care
	Association work

Source: American Society of Health-System Pharmacists. Required and elective outcomes, goals, objectives, and instructional objectives for postgraduate year one (PGY1) pharmacy residency programs, 2nd edition—effective July 2008. http://www.ashp.org/DocLibrary/Accreditation/PGY1-Goals-Objectives.aspx. Accessed March 31, 2011. Reprinted with permission.

in electives. Typically, at the beginning of the residency year, the experiences are individualized to meet the goals of the resident.

Community pharmacy residents are primarily responsible for direct patient care, practice management, teaching, and project management. **Table 4-2** provides examples of resident responsibilities and activities. Community residents spend the majority of their time providing patient care activities.

Direct patient care may include the provision of medication therapy management, disease state management and education,

> **Community residents spend the majority of their time providing patient care activities.**

prevention and wellness screening, immunization administration, and group education. Community pharmacy residents may also spend time in ambulatory care clinics providing patient care services in collaboration with other healthcare providers. Community residents are responsible for developing, implementing, and evaluating new patient care services. Residents have implemented services such as immunizations, anticoagulation management, smoking cessation, and diabetes education. As part of this process, residents learn how to write a business plan. They gain experience in marketing, compensation, and management. As in other residencies, community pharmacy residents are responsible for developing and conducting a project during the residency year. Community pharmacy residents have opportunities for teaching student pharmacists, patients, caregivers, and other healthcare professionals. Many community pharmacy residency programs offer teaching certificates upon successful completion of the residency. Residents can usually choose electives, which can be used to enhance learning experiences by delving more deeply into one or more areas of interest or gaining exposure to other areas of interest. Table 4-1 lists elective outcomes of the ASHP–APhA accreditation standard.

CHOOSING A COMMUNITY PHARMACY RESIDENCY PROGRAM

Student pharmacists should seriously consider choosing a community pharmacy residency that is accredited by ASHP–APhA. Accreditation ensures that the residency program meets a required standard for education and training. Other factors to consider include the college or school of pharmacy affiliation, geographic location, number of sites within the program, and training opportunities. Student pharmacists should consider the focus of the residency program, which should align with the student pharmacist's career goals. The APhA website (www.pharmacist.com) has a list of questions that a resident can use when evaluating community pharmacy residency programs.

COMMUNITY PHARMACY RESIDENTS IN PRACTICE

Community pharmacy residents have multiple options for positions after graduation: traditional dispensing with dedicated time for other patient care activities, full-time patient care activities, clinical coordinator, and manager. Some graduates work toward pharmacy ownership or are current pharmacy owners. Other residency graduates take faculty positions, often sharing their time between a community pharmacy site and a school or college of pharmacy. Some community residents provide patient care in ambulatory care clinics, whereas others serve as consultants for nontraditional pharmacy settings.

Community pharmacy residency graduates are well educated and trained for a career in innovative community practice.

Beyond their job, community pharmacy residency graduates are engaged in the profession and the community. Anecdotally, this author has observed that past community pharmacy residency graduates actively seek to serve the profession by volunteering for committees and holding offices in local, state, and national organizations at a high rate. Community pharmacy residency graduates are well educated and trained for a career in innovative community practice. They are also well prepared for a multitude of positions and opportunities.

KEY POINTS

- Student pharmacists should consider a PGY1 community pharmacy residency if they wish to focus on high-level, direct patient care in this setting.

- PGY1 community pharmacy residencies have the same rigor and standards as other PGY1 residencies.

- Choosing a PGY1 community pharmacy residency is based on the program's structure, accreditation status, longitudinal experiences, and program mentors.

- Community pharmacy residencies provide a variety of experiences and prepare graduates to lead practice change.

- Those completing a community pharmacy residency have multiple options: dedicated patient care, leadership (clinical coordinator or manager), pharmacy ownership, and faculty positions.

REFERENCES

1. American Society of Health-System Pharmacists. Pharmacy residency training in the future: a stakeholders' roundtable discussion. *Am J Health Sys Pharm.* 2005;62:1817–1820.
2. American Pharmacists Association. Community pharmacy residency program accreditation. http://www.pharmacist.com/AM/Template.cfm?Section=Residencies_Advanced_Training&TEMPLATE=/CM/HTMLDisplay.cfm&CONTENTID=3028. Accessed March 31, 2011.
3. Schommer JC, Bonnarens JK, Brown LB, Goode JR. Value of community pharmacy residency programs: college of pharmacy and practice site perceptions. *J Am Pharm Assoc.* 2010;50:e72–e88.
4. Unterwagner WL, Zeolla MM, Burns AL. Training experiences of current and former community pharmacy residents, 1986–2000. *J Am Pharm Assoc.* 2003;43:201–206.
5. American Society of Health-System Pharmacists, American Pharmacists Association. Accreditation standard for postgraduate year one (PGY1) community pharmacy residency programs. http://www.ashp.org/DocLibrary/Accreditation/ASD-PGY1-Community-Standard.aspx. Accessed March 31, 2011.
6. American Society of Health-System Pharmacists. ASHP accreditation standard for postgraduate year one (PGY1) pharmacy residency programs. http://www.ashp.org/s_ashp/docs/files/RTP_PGY1AccredStandard.pdf. Accessed March 31, 2011.

CHAPTER 5

Postgraduate Year One (PGY1) Managed Care Pharmacy Residency Programs

Rusty Hailey and Annie M. Rakoczy

Action is the foundational key to all successes.

—Pablo Picasso

QUESTIONS TO PONDER

1. What is managed care pharmacy, and why is it important?

2. What training experiences may a resident complete during a managed care residency program?

3. What career options are available for managed care pharmacy residency program graduates?

4. Where can a residency applicant learn more about available programs and the application process?

Managed care is an approach to deliver healthcare services that puts scarce resources to the best use to optimize patient care.[1] For more than a century, managed care initiatives have made a significant impact on the U.S. healthcare delivery system. As managed care organizations (MCOs) balance the cost and quality of care delivered to patients, managed care principles have driven the ability to attain cost-effective, high-quality care. Pharmacists play key roles in many of these initiatives, including health and wellness, disease prevention, coordination of care, and utilization management.

> **Managed care is an approach to deliver healthcare services that puts scarce resources to the best use.**

Managed care principles that assist in achieving this balance include, but are not limited to, prior authorizations, drug utilization reviews, outcomes research, prescription benefit management, and specialty pharmaceutical therapy management. For instance, by actively maintaining a formulary for a prescription drug benefit, a team of pharmacists, physicians, and other healthcare professionals promote cost-effective therapies, improve access to more affordable care, and decrease medical costs and hospitalization rates. Therefore, managed care principles are put in place for reasons that include the containment of rising healthcare premiums, management of off-label indications of therapy not supported by evidence-based literature, monitoring the amount of medication dispensed over a period of time, and alerting a pharmacy to quantities above a daily safety limit.

Although the impact of managed care can be experienced in the community and hospital settings, survey results and related focus groups suggest that student pharmacists feel uninformed about managed care.[2]

> A managed care pharmacy residency can be a valuable opportunity to gain further understanding of what managed care entails.

Consequently, a managed care pharmacy residency can be a valuable opportunity to gain further understanding of what managed care entails. It can provide the experiences and knowledge that will position a pharmacy resident for a career in the managed care industry. As the United States encounters rising healthcare expenditures, increased life expectancies, and legislation providing health insurance to a greater portion of the population, there will continue to be a need for pharmacists in managed care fields to contribute to the essential services that will balance the cost and quality of care delivered.

OUTCOMES AND EXPERIENCES

Existing accreditation standards for managed care pharmacy residencies are determined jointly by the American Society of Health-System Pharmacists (ASHP) and the Academy of Managed Care Pharmacy (AMCP) for managed care postgraduate year one (PGY1) programs; however, not all managed care pharmacy residencies are accredited programs. The ASHP–AMCP accreditation standards for PGY1 managed care pharmacy residency programs establish the criteria for systematic training of pharmacists for achieving professional competence in the delivery of patient-centered care and in pharmacy operational services in managed care settings.[3] Residents must achieve similar outcome competencies to other ASHP PGY1 programs. **Table 5-1** compares the outcomes of a PGY1 Managed Care Pharmacy Residency with the PGY1 Pharmacy Residency.[3,4] Unique to PGY1 managed care programs are required outcomes related to the drug distribution process for organization members and the design of effective benefit structures.

A resident may work with the corporate leadership of a healthcare plan to analyze different benefit structures to offer their membership, review how a pharmacy contracts with a pharmacy benefit manager (PBM), write

Table 5-1 Comparison of Educational Outcomes Between PGY1 Managed Care Pharmacy Residency Programs and PGY1 Pharmacy Residency Programs

PGY1 Managed Care Pharmacy Residency Programs	PGY1 Pharmacy Residency Programs
Required Outcomes (Matched by Content)	
Outcome R1: Understand how to manage the drug distribution process for an organization's members.	
Outcome R2: Design and implement clinical programs to enhance the efficacy of patient care.	Outcome R2: Provide evidence-based, patient-centered medication therapy management with interdisciplinary teams.
Outcome R3: Ensure the safety and quality of the medication-use system.	Outcome R1: Manage and improve the medication-use process.
Outcome R4: Provide medication and practice-related information, education, and/or training.	Outcome R5: Provide medication and practice-related education and training.
Outcome R5: Collaborate with plan sponsors to design effective benefit structures to service a specific population's needs.	
Outcome R6: Exercise leadership and practice management skills.	Outcome R3: Exercise leadership and practice management skills.
Outcome R7: Demonstrate project management skills.	Outcome R4: Demonstrate project management skills.
	Outcome R6: Utilize medical informatics.
Elective Outcomes (Matched by Content)	
Outcome E1: Added knowledge and skills to manage the drug distribution process for the organization's members.	
Outcome E2: Provide evidence-based, patient-centered medication therapy management with interdisciplinary teams.	
Outcome E3: Added knowledge and skills to provide medication and practice-related information, education, and/or training.	

Table 5-1 Comparison of Educational Outcomes Between PGY1 Managed Care Pharmacy Residency Programs and PGY1 Pharmacy Residency Programs (*Continued*)

PGY1 Managed Care Pharmacy Residency Programs	*PGY1 Pharmacy Residency Programs*
Outcome E4: Exercise added leadership and practice management skills.	Outcome E2: Exercise added leadership and practice management skills.
Outcome E5: Participate in the process by which managed care organizations contract with pharmaceutical manufacturers.	
Outcome E6: Conduct outcomes-based research.	
Outcome E7: Conduct pharmacy practice research.	Outcome E1: Conduct pharmacy practice research.
Outcome E8: Participate in the management of business continuity.	
Outcome E9: Demonstrate additional competencies that contribute to working successfully in the healthcare environment.	Outcome E7: Demonstrate additional competencies that contribute to working successfully in the healthcare environment.
	Outcome E3: Demonstrate knowledge and skills particular to generalist practice in the home care practice environment.
	Outcome E4: Demonstrate knowledge and skills particular to generalist practice in the managed care practice environment.
	Outcome E5: Participate in the management of medical emergencies.
	Outcome E6: Provide drug information to healthcare professionals and/or the public.

Sources: Modified from American Society of Health-System Pharmacists, Academy of Managed Care Pharmacy. Required and elective educational outcomes, educational goals, educational objectives, and instructional objectives for postgraduate year one (PGY1) managed care pharmacy residency programs. http://www.ashp.org/DocLibrary/Accreditation/RTPManagedCare-Goals-and-Objective-Criteria2010.aspx. Accessed March 31, 2011. Reprinted with permission; and American Society of Health-System Pharmacists. Required and elective educational outcomes, goals, objectives, and instructional objectives for postgraduate year one (PGY1) pharmacy residency programs, 2nd edition—effective July 2008. http://www.ashp.org/DocLibrary/Accreditation/PGY1-Goals-Objectives.aspx. Accessed March 31, 2011. Reprinted with permission.

drug monographs and prior authorization criteria for a pharmacy and therapeutics (P&T) committee, and develop a pharmacy quality initiative after analyzing pharmacy claims data. These activities may consist of short-term rotations, longitudinal rotations, or experiences that span a period of months.

RESIDENCY PROGRAMS

Common settings for managed care residencies include health plans, PBM organizations, and health maintenance organizations (HMOs). Residencies may have a partnership with a local school or college of pharmacy, allowing the residents to improve their teaching skills. These organizations expose residents to diverse patient populations, complex patient issues, a variety of medication therapy management techniques, and clinical programs designed for both large populations and individual patients. Residents may fulfill similar job responsibilities to those of pharmacists within the organization, such as completing prior authorizations, conducting medication therapy management (MTM) reviews, counseling patients, and developing criteria for the drug utilization review (DUR) program. Oftentimes, program leaders have completed a residency and thus recognize the value of providing residency training to the future of the profession. Not infrequently, organizations recruit residents for internal open positions at the conclusion of their 12-month training period. As a result, a residency can be a win–win for both the resident and the program; the resident earns a position after completion, and the site has a year to evaluate the skill level, interest, and commitment of the resident.

> Common settings for managed care residencies include health plans, PBM organizations, and health maintenance organizations (HMOs).

Depending on the program's unique configuration, clinical pharmacists, pharmacy managers, clinical program directors, or chief pharmacy officers may serve in the roles of residency program director, coordinator, or preceptor. These individuals may be employed in a particular department of the company and may hold titles such as analytic consulting services consultant, specialty pharmacy services manager, and clinical pharmacy director. The variety of services an organization provides to its members expands the practice skills of the resident and provides unique interactions with other healthcare professionals throughout the year. For residency candidates who value learning from a variety of preceptors and want to gain a deeper understanding of an assortment of managed care principles, it is advantageous to choose sites that offer services to a larger population base.

> The variety of services an organization provides to its members expands the practice skills of the resident and provides unique interactions with other healthcare professionals throughout the year.

The knowledge gained by a resident will vary by site and whether the program is accredited or not; however, during the year a resident may be required to do the following:

- Explain what impact the maximum allowable cost (MAC) of drugs has within a health plan.

- Demonstrate how companies bill through an online claims adjudication system.

- Determine whether a new therapy should be presented to a P&T committee as cost-effective in comparison to existing therapies.

- Incorporate utilization management (UM) tools into a formulary.

- Design a medication therapy management program for a particular patient population.

- Explain how an organization provides specialty pharmacy services.

- Describe how quality improvement plans are incorporated; describe ways that an organization can improve their Healthcare Effectiveness Data and Information Set (HEDIS) measures.

An example of a non-patient-care activity in a health plan is a rebate contracting rotation. During the rotation, the resident works with the rebate team to understand the process for contracting with pharmaceutical manufacturers. In learning why contracts between the two parties exist, the resident may be involved in various meetings reviewing contracts and demonstrating how the formulary placement of a drug complies with a contract. The resident may have to prepare periodic financial models signifying the impact of a rebate proposal within a class of drugs for a disease state. This involves understanding the market share of a drug and the utilization of drugs within a market basket.

Most residents in a managed care residency complete a residency project, as they would do in other PGY1 programs. Since many managed care programs have access to large amounts of pharmacy and/or medical claims data, residents are uniquely positioned to analyze utilization patterns and develop suggestions to either better manage a disease state or to change a benefit structure.

> The experiences available to managed care residents allow for a variety of positions at an array of different practice sites.

The experiences available to managed care residents allow for a variety of positions at an array of different practice sites upon program completion. Managed care residency alumni hold positions within a variety of companies, such as HMOs, Veterans Affairs medical centers, pharmaceutical companies, Medicare Advantage Plans, MTM vendors, and consulting firms. Often residency alumni start as clinical staff pharmacists and move up the leadership chain, applying leadership skills learned during the residency program. Although a residency is not a requirement for all clinical staff pharmacists in managed care positions, some companies require a residency or a certain number of years of clinical pharmacy experience. With every earned success, residents increase their chances of becoming managers, directors, and even presidents of companies. Beginning by completing a residency that gains exposure to different managed care principles, a career as a clinical managed care staff pharmacist can be attained by talented pharmacists in managed care pharmacy.

RESIDENCY CHOICES

Both the ASHP and AMCP post a partial listing of managed care pharmacy residencies available throughout the country on their websites. These sites provide contact information for program leadership so that individuals wishing to apply for residencies can inquire about the program requirements and obtain applications. Many residency programs attend the ASHP (annually in December) and/or AMCP (annually in April) conferences. These opportunities allow residents to speak personally with representatives of the various residency programs, including current residents, without investing the time and money to travel to each interview. The AMCP Managed Care Pharmacy Residency Showcase attracts a large number of managed care pharmacy residencies and candidates. As a result, prospective residents may find that this interactive venue, due to its intimate setting, allows them to spend time with key individuals from the available programs prior to applying.

The ASHP Midyear Clinical Meeting allows candidates to interview for managed care residency programs. As with other PGY1 programs, residencies seeking accreditation, as well as those that are accredited, participate in the ASHP Residency Matching Program. The nonaccredited programs list the program application deadline on the AMCP website and may secure positions prior to the match. Some residencies require essays, letters of recommendation, or on-site interviews, so candidates should carefully review the requirements for each program.

RESIDENCY CANDIDATES

If a residency candidate is not familiar with the basic managed care principles, the AMCP website offers articles explaining managed care terminology and describing how the concepts are implemented in a managed care setting.[5] In addition, the student center webpage within the website provides resources, such as PowerPoint presentations, that address the issues and concepts in everyday managed care practice settings. Before completing the application and interviewing for a managed care residency, candidates should adequately prepare, using resources such as these, to become familiar with managed care pharmacy. Candidates also should be prepared to discuss and clarify their reasons for seeking a residency program in this

> If a residency candidate is not familiar with the basic managed care principles, the AMCP website offers articles explaining managed care terminology and describing how the concepts are implemented in a managed care setting.

particular field. This will help candidates write a more informed and relevant application and be better prepared to answer questions from the interviewers. Understanding how managed care issues directly affect a program setting will also allow candidates to compose relevant questions to demonstrate their eagerness to learn and their interest in managed care pharmacy.

Although program settings vary, many are in corporate environments that are timeline driven, project based, and do not have an on-site pharmacy. Some programs have rotations in the residency whereby residents communicate with patients over the phone, face to face, or both. Understanding that the environment may be different from other experiences will assist the resident in adapting to some settings that are office based. Many programs look for candidates who can adapt to an office setting, do not need daily patient contact, understand basic managed care principles, and are eager to utilize the clinical knowledge they gained in pharmacy school to balance the cost and quality of care being delivered.

Candidates interested in a managed care pharmacy residency should understand how it differs from other PGY1 programs. For example, the delivery of patient-centered care in a managed care setting involves pharmacy services that apply principles such as utilization management. Likewise, the outcomes and experiences may be different, and the resident may be involved in committees with the corporate leadership of a health plan analyzing different benefit structures to offer the plan membership. Nevertheless, all of the differences can be exciting, and they open many doors for residents in careers in a growing healthcare field, such as specialty pharmacy and pharmacy benefit management. To learn more, candidates are encouraged to become active in pharmacy organizations, including AMCP, whereby they can become familiar with the application process, network with residency program leaders at conferences, and understand how current managed care issues directly affect a program setting.

> Candidates interested in a managed care pharmacy residency should understand how it differs from other PGY1 programs.

As the field of managed care continues to balance cost efficiency with quality of care, pharmacists will play an essential role in reaching this balance and improving patient outcomes. Through coordinated healthcare delivery, management of resource utilization, preventive care benefit services, and disease management programs, managed care residency programs offer an opportunity for interested candidates to gain knowledge in the field while positioning them for any number of careers in the managed care industry. Considering that "action is the foundational key to all successes," taking the first step and completing a managed care pharmacy residency will position a pharmacist for a successful career.

KEY POINTS

- Managed care principles that assist in achieving a balance of cost and quality of care include, but are not limited to, prior authorizations, drug utilization reviews, outcomes research, prescription benefits management, and specialty pharmaceutical therapy management.

- Unique to the PGY1 managed care program are required outcomes related to the drug distribution process for organization members and the design of effective benefit structures.

- The AMCP Managed Care Pharmacy Residency Showcase includes a number of managed care pharmacy residencies and is an interactive venue that allows candidates time to interact with key individuals from programs before applying.

- To best prepare, residency candidates are encouraged to learn about the practice of managed care pharmacy, including reviewing information from the AMCP student center and talking to managed care pharmacists.

- Managed care residency alumni hold positions within a variety of companies, such as HMOs, Veterans Affairs medical centers, pharmaceutical companies, Medicare Advantage Plans, MTM vendors, and consulting firms.

REFERENCES

1. Novarro RP, Cahill JA. Role of managed care in the US healthcare system. In: Novarro RP, ed. *Managed Care Pharmacy Practice*. Sudbury, MA: Jones and Bartlett Publishers; 2009:1.
2. Pittenger A, Starner C, Thompson K, Gleason P. Pharmacy students' views of managed care pharmacy and PBMs: should there be more exposure to managed care in the pharmacy curriculum? *J Manag Care Pharm.* 2010;16(5):346–354.
3. American Society of Health-System Pharmacists, Academy of Managed Care Pharmacy. Accreditation standard for postgraduate year one (PGY1) managed care pharmacy residency programs. http://www.ashp.org/DocLibrary/Accreditation/ASD-Managed-Care-Standard.aspx. Accessed March 31, 2011.
4. American Society of Health-System Pharmacists. ASHP accreditation standard for postgraduate year one (PGY1) pharmacy practice residency programs. http://www.ashp.org/DocLibrary/Accreditation/ASD-PGY1-Standard.aspx. Accessed March 31, 2011.
5. Academy of Managed Care Pharmacy. Residencies. http://www.amcp.org/amcp.ark?p=AAF027AF. Accessed March 31, 2011.

CHAPTER 6

Ambulatory-Based Residencies

L. Brian Cross

I never teach my pupils; I only attempt to provide the conditions in which they can learn.

—Albert Einstein

QUESTIONS TO PONDER

1. What is ambulatory care?

2. Will an ambulatory care residency meet the applicant's practice and career goals?

3. What training experiences should one expect in an ambulatory care residency?

4. What qualities differentiate one ambulatory care residency from another?

The American College of Clinical Pharmacy (ACCP), the American Pharmacists Association (APhA), and the American Society of Health-System Pharmacists (ASHP), in their 2001 petition to the Board of Pharmaceutical Specialties (BPS) requesting recognition of ambulatory care pharmacy practice as a specialty, define ambulatory care as "The provision of integrated, accessible healthcare services by pharmacists who are accountable for addressing medication needs, developing sustained partnerships with patients, and practicing in the context of family and community."[1]

The petition also states that ambulatory care pharmacy practice is "Accomplished through direct patient care and medication management for ambulatory patients, long-term relationships, coordination of care, patient advocacy, wellness and health promotion, triage and referral, and patient education and self-management."[1]

Healthcare continues to move toward preventing hospitalization and focusing on the primary care model of medicine or patient-centered medical home. The recent passage of the Patient Protection and Affordable Care Act and the Health Care and Education Reconciliation Act of 2010 has stimulated a growing interest in better management of the complicated medication regimens of potentially millions of newly insured patients with multiple chronic medical conditions. This seems to be a perfect symbiotic relationship in the making: a dearth of clinical services being provided for a significantly increasing number of patients and a desire of well-trained practitioners to step forward and fill that void. Hopefully, this will result in a significantly increased engagement of clinical pharmacy practitioners in the ambulatory setting.

> **Healthcare continues to move toward preventing hospitalization and focusing on the primary care model of medicine.**

With this changing healthcare environment as the backdrop, candidates considering an ambulatory-based residency must assess how this potential training will enable them to be directly responsible for patient medication management while being incorporated into a team-based approach to care.

• Longitudinal Versus Episodic Versus Continuity Care

Some differences among potential ambulatory care sites for residency training are based in the manner, and sometimes in the settings, in which care is provided. Some programs provide all patient care and residency training in the ambulatory setting. This environment will often provide learning experiences that are both longitudinal (caring for the same group of patients over an extended period) and episodic (seeing unique groups of patients for a short period) in nature. However, some ambulatory care residency programs expose trainees to acute care inpatient environments. In these continuity care training settings, the resident gains experience following patients as they travel from acute inpatient settings, to rehabilitation settings, to ambulatory clinic settings, and back. This level of continuity of care most commonly characterizes family-medicine-based training programs. Both of these approaches to ambulatory care pharmacy practice have strengths and weaknesses; therefore, prospective residents should attempt to match their educational and practice objectives to the setting and focus of the training programs they are evaluating.

• Disease Management Versus Pharmacotherapy Management

An issue requiring brief discussion is how the program is focused. The two models most commonly seen in ambulatory pharmacy practice settings are disease-management-based clinics (e.g., diabetes, heart failure, anticoagulation, hypertension, and lipids) and pharmacotherapy-management-based clinics (e.g. pharmaceutical care clinic and medication management clinic). In disease-management-based clinics, pharmacists are often responsible for the direct care of patients with certain chronic diseases, such as diabetes, hypertension, hyperlipidemia, heart failure, chronic antico-agulation, smoking cessation, asthma, COPD, HIV/AIDS, or chronic pain. This approach to care provides a focused exposure on chronic care issues and often places the pharmacist in the center of management issues. One survey reported that the most common areas of practice for pharmacists in ambula-tory settings were anticoagulation therapy (36%), oncology (28%), primary care and family medicine (23%), diabetes (21%), HIV infection and AIDS (17%), and medication management (16%).[2] Many pharmacy practitioners often acquire additional credentialing specific to the chronic disease(s) with which they most commonly work, such as diabetes (CDE and BC-ADM), lipids (CLS), anticoagulation (CACP), asthma (AE-C), HIV (AAHIVE), geriatrics (CGP), pain management (DAAPM), or women's health issues (NCMP). In pharmacotherapy-management-based clinics, pharmacists are often involved more holistically in the overall assessment and management of patients' entire medication regimens. The continued focus on medication therapy management (MTM) and the more recent spotlight on the patient-centered medical home (PCMH) will continue to reinforce the importance of pharmacist involvement in pharmacotherapy-management-based clinics. Regardless of the focus of the potential practice site (disease focused versus pharmacotherapy focused), the residency candidate should be aware of the level of practice allowed based on practice acts in the given state of training, as well as through collaborative prac-tice agreements and scope of practice documents with the prac-tice site. These agreements will provide insight into the level of practice at which the resident will potentially be engaged during his or her training. Prospective residents should consider which model (disease or pharmacotherapy management) more closely mirrors their training goals and will best prepare them for the type of practice they desire in the future.

> Prospective residents should consider which model (disease or pharmacotherapy management) more closely mirrors their training goals.

NATIONAL PHARMACY ORGANIZATIONS' VIEWS ON AMBULATORY CARE

• American Association of Colleges of Pharmacy (AACP)

In the most recent report of AACP's Argus Commission, a significant emphasis was placed on the importance of expanding pharmacy's role in primary care settings.[3] This document heightened awareness of the need for relevant primary care competencies in both the curricula of colleges and schools of pharmacy and in national licensure examinations. The docu-ment also highlighted the need for increased interprofessional education experiences that better incorporate the pharmacist as a vital player on the healthcare team. Lastly, the document strongly recommends the need for the development of a plan to achieve uniform national regulation for pharmacists' patient care activities.

• American College of Clinical Pharmacy (ACCP)

Recent publications from ACCP have called for both residency training and board certification as a prerequisite for a pharmacist's involvement in direct patient care.[4,5] In addition, they also recommend that all residency programs be accredited as either a postgraduate year one (PGY1) or postgraduate year two (PGY2) residency and that PGY1 residency training be a minimal requirement for academic appointment as an adjunct clinical faculty member or preceptor. The organization also suggests that all PGY2 residencies require previous completion of a PGY1 residency, though advanced practice residencies may be offered as two-year programs in which general pharmacy practice (PGY1) training is the major focus of the first year. The ACCP urges that instruction in teaching methods be made available to residents as part of their overall training and that new full-time clinician–educator faculty appointed to the rank of assistant professor should have completed at least two years of postgraduate residency training. The publication of these guidelines, combined with the aforementioned petition to the BPS to recognize ambulatory care pharmacy practice as a specialty with a corresponding board certification exam, suggest that a more structured, consistent definition of ambulatory care will prevail in the future. It remains to be seen how this certification versus other disease-specific credentials will be utilized in ambulatory care pharmacy practice in the future, as well as whether ambulatory care residencies will be considered preparatory for this certification in the same way pharmacotherapy residencies are for the BCPS examination. It should be noted that recent eligibility criteria for the ambulatory care pharmacy practice exam published by the BPS states that candidates must have gained four years of practice experience in ambulatory care pharmacy activities (at least 50% of time in ambulatory care), or completed a PGY1 residency plus one year of experience in ambulatory care pharmacy activities (at least 50% of time in ambulatory care), or completed a PGY2 residency in ambulatory care. Furthermore, the criteria will accept candidates only from ASHP-accredited residencies (PGY1 and PGY2) after January 1, 2013.[6]

• American Society of Health-System Pharmacists (ASHP)

The ASHP Educational Outcomes, Goals, and Objectives for Postgraduate Year Two (PGY2) Ambulatory Care Pharmacy Residency Programs clearly outline the required outcomes for trainees completing a PGY2 residency in ambulatory care.[7] These outcomes, categorized by required and elective, are provided in **Table 6-1**.

The ASHP outcomes document clearly suggests a desire for ambulatory care residency training to be a PGY2 specialty that prepares trainees to be part of a collaborative care team,

> The ASHP outcomes document clearly suggests a desire for ambulatory care residency training to be a PGY2 specialty.

Table 6-1 Educational Outcomes for PGY2 Ambulatory Care Pharmacy Residency Programs

Required Outcomes

Outcome R1:	Establish a collaborative interdisciplinary practice.
Outcome R2:	In a collaborative interdisciplinary ambulatory practice, provide efficient, effective, evidence-based, patient-centered treatment for chronic and/or acute illnesses in all degrees of complexity.
Outcome R3:	Demonstrate leadership and practice management skills.
Outcome R4:	Promote health improvement, wellness, and disease prevention.
Outcome R5:	Demonstrate excellence in the provision of training or educational activities for healthcare professionals and healthcare professionals in training.
Outcome R6:	Serve as an authoritative resource on the optimal use of medications.

Elective Outcomes

Outcome E1:	When the ambulatory pharmacy practice is within a setting that allows pharmacist credentialing, successfully apply for credentialing.
Outcome E2:	Understand the role of the ambulatory care pharmacy leader in the development of public health policy.
Outcome E3:	Participate in the management of medical emergencies.
Outcome E4:	When the practice includes integrated care, such as in family medicine, provide efficient, effective, evidence-based, patient-centered treatment for chronic and/or acute illnesses in all degrees of complexity to hospitalized patients.
Outcome E5:	Demonstrate skills required to function in an academic setting.

Source: Modified from American Society of Health-System Pharmacists. Educational outcomes, goals, and objectives for postgraduate year two (PGY2) ambulatory care pharmacy residency programs. http://www.ashp.org/s_ashp/docs/files/accreditation/RTP_ObjAmbulatory032608. doc. Accessed March 31, 2011. Reprinted with permission.

a leader in practice management issues, a drug therapy authority, and possibly a candidate prepared for future credentialing processes, as well as a highly functioning academician. Pharmacy graduates considering an ambulatory care residency should determine whether potential programs can provide this level of training.

PRACTICE SITES FOR AMBULATORY-BASED RESIDENCY PROGRAMS

Ambulatory care residencies exist in varied settings across the healthcare spectrum. Ambulatory care pharmacists are involved in multiple health-system settings including community hospitals, integrated health networks or HMOs, teaching institutions, federally sponsored facilities, and Veterans Affairs (VA) medical centers.[3] Today, ambulatory care residencies can be found in the following settings:

- Government facilities, such as the VA and Indian Health Service
- Safety-net-type clinics, such as community health clinics (CHCs)
- Federally-qualified health centers (FQHCs) and area health education centers (AHECs)
- Large closed healthcare systems, such as Kaiser Permanente and Intermountain Healthcare
- Family medicine residency teaching programs
- Private practice medical groups

Each type of practice site has strengths and weaknesses, which the prospective resident should attempt to correlate with his or her individual educational goals.

• The Value of PGY1 and PGY2 Residencies in Ambulatory Care

As discussed previously, strong recommendations from multiple national pharmacy organizations (AACP, ACCP, and ASHP) are beginning to converge, establishing a consensus that pharmacists delivering direct patient care must obtain at least one residency and board certification. Some colleges and schools of pharmacy prefer a second year of residency training for faculty appointments. Any specialized residency-training program will be required to receive accreditation as a PGY2 program. This is clearly the global direction of professional education in pharmacy; however, when one compares the ASHP residency directory[8] to the ACCP residency directory[9] for listings describing training programs in ambulatory or primary care, more than 50% of listings in the ACCP directory are described as PGY1 programs. Oftentimes these programs are self-described as having a "focus" or "emphasis" in ambulatory care. The clear perceived advantage from the trainee's perspective is the ability to obtain training in ambulatory care in one year without having to complete a general pharmacy practice residency (PGY1) followed by a subsequent PGY2 residency in ambulatory care; however, it is important to note the missed training opportunities and potential implications for future training options and career choices that may exist with this model. First, some may argue that the trainee is receiving neither a full, broad

PGY1 experience nor an advanced PGY2 experience focusing on ambulatory care. Second, trends in training suggest that advanced pharmacy practitioners in ambulatory care will eventually be required to have completed a PGY2 residency as well as be board certified. Completing a PGY1 residency with emphasis in ambulatory care may limit potential employment options for the trainee later in his or her career. Again, the resident's choice of programs should align with his or her future professional goals.

> Completing a PGY1 residency with emphasis in ambulatory care may limit potential employment options.

• Roles and Responsibilities

Potential trainees should understand how any residency program they are considering is structured and what unique roles and responsibilities the program entails, in order to make an informed decision. Issues to clarify include inpatient care responsibilities; the focus of the clinic, whether disease state, pharmacotherapy, or a hybrid; level of practice allowed based on collaborative agreements of the clinic's resident staff; and level of incorporation into an interprofessional team of patient care.

• Level of College or School of Pharmacy Involvement

Residency graduates seeking acceptance with a college of pharmacy as an ambulatory faculty member should determine what level of teaching involvement would be required in collaboration with nearby colleges of pharmacy. Many residency programs are now incorporating teaching and learning certificates into residency training to help prepare the trainee for a smoother transition into a possible full-time faculty appointment with a college of pharmacy. If this is a path a candidate for residency foresees taking, it may be important to ask potential residency programs if a teaching and learning certificate is available.

KEY POINTS

- Candidates for training in ambulatory care residency programs should choose a program that allows them to focus on specific expectations.

- Practice settings in ambulatory care vary based on specific patient populations, disease states of interest, integration within an interdisciplinary team, and involvement in academia.

- Training programs in ambulatory care should make trainees competent, autonomous providers of direct patient care in multidisciplinary practice environments, as well as prepare them to pursue specialty credentialing as required for future practice.

REFERENCES

1. Brennan C, Goode JVR, Haines S, et al. A petition to the Board of Pharmaceutical Specialties requesting recognition of ambulatory care pharmacy practice as a specialty. http://www.accp.com/docs/positions/petitions/BPS_Ambulatory_Care_Petition.pdf. Accessed March 31, 2011.

2. Knapp KK, Okamoto MP, Black BL. ASHP survey of ambulatory care pharmacy practice in health systems 2004. *Am J Health Syst Pharm*. 2005;62:274–284.

3. American Association of Colleges of Pharmacy Argus Committee. Call to action: expansion of pharmacy primary care services in a reformed health system. www .aacp.org/GOVERNANCE/COMMITTEES/ARGUS/Pages/CommitteeReports .aspx. Accessed March 31, 2011.

4. Murphy JE, Nappi JM, Bosso JA, et al. American College of Clinical Pharmacy's vision of the future: postgraduate pharmacy residency training as a prerequisite for direct patient care practice. *Pharmacotherapy*. 2006;26:722–733.

5. Saseen JJ, Grady SE, Hansen LB, et al. American College of Clinical Pharmacy white paper: future clinical pharmacy practitioners should be board-certified specialists. *Pharmacotherapy*. 2006;26:1816–1825.

6. Board of Pharmacy Specialties. Specialties: ambulatory care. www.bpsweb.org/ specialties/AmbulatoryCarePharmacy.cfm. Accessed March 31, 2011.

7. American Society of Health-System Pharmacists. Educational outcomes, goals, and objectives for postgraduate year two (PGY2) ambulatory care pharmacy residency programs. http://www.ashp.org/s_ashp/docs/files/accreditation/RTP_ ObjAmbulatory032608.doc. Accessed March 31, 2011.

8. American Society of Health-System Pharmacists. Residency directory. http:// www.ashp.org/Import/ACCREDITATION/ResidencyDirectory.aspx. Accessed March 31, 2011.

9. American College of Clinical Pharmacy. Directory of residencies, fellowships, and graduate programs. www.accp.com/resandfel/search.aspx. Accessed March 31, 2011.

CHAPTER 7

Postgraduate Year Two (PGY2) Pharmacy Residency Programs

Brian L. Erstad

Two roads diverged in a yellow wood, And sorry I could not travel both

— from "The Road Not Taken" by Robert Frost

QUESTIONS TO PONDER

1. Does the postgraduate year two (PGY2) applicant have a passion for an area of specialization and desire to focus his or her professional career in that area?

2. Is the PGY2 applicant excited about a particular area of specialization because of positive experiences in that area or because of a passion independent of personnel?

3. Is the PGY2 applicant aware of the range of experiences available in PGY2 programs under consideration?

4. Based on all of the subjective and objective information regarding a program and program director, does the applicant believe that there is a good match?

5. Is the applicant aware of the potential advantages and disadvantages associated with the early commitment process?

The intent of this chapter is to provide some relevant considerations for prospective residents attempting to secure and subsequently excel in a

PGY2 program. Most of the focus will be on explaining the options for PGY2 training and methods to secure a program.

HISTORICAL PERSPECTIVE

It is difficult to pinpoint the date when specialized pharmacy residencies first came into existence, but specialization began to flourish in the late 1980s and early 1990s after the publication of accreditation standards for specialized pharmacy residency training in 1980 by the American Society of Health-System Pharmacists (ASHP, known as the American Society of Hospital Pharmacists at the time).[1] In conjunction with the publication of the accreditation standards for specialized pharmacy residency training, a supplementary standard and learning objectives for residencies in psychiatric pharmacy practice was also released.[2] The first revision of the specialized pharmacy residency training standard was published in 1988.[3] When the second revision was published in 1994, there were supplemental standards for oncology and drug information in addition to psychopharmacy.[4] During the ensuing years, a good deal of discussion took place concerning the definition of a *specialty*. This led to the release of accreditation standards in 2005 that addressed general versus specialized residency training. (See Chapter 1, "Introduction to Postgraduate Training Opportunities," for a description and comparison.)

From a terminology standpoint, pharmacy residencies are now defined as postgraduate year one (PGY1) and postgraduate year two (PGY2). Additionally, residency programs listed as specialized at the time, but arguably could be considered general or specialty (e.g., primary care, pediatrics), were given the option of becoming PGY1 or PGY2 programs by the 2007 to 2008 residency year, with the caveat that the programs train residents in the applicable outcomes.[5] Prior to 2007, specialized residences were not required to participate in the Residency Matching Program, but along with the new PGY1–PGY2 classification appeared a condition that all programs accredited by ASHP enter the match. (See Chapter 16, "The Residency Matching Program," for more information). Additionally, PGY2 program directors are required to obtain board certification in available areas.[6]

OPTIONS FOR PGY2 TRAINING

By 2011, numerous types of PGY2 residencies were listed on the ASHP accreditation website (see **Table 7-1**). Although it can be argued that all pharmacists specialize to some degree, a quick review of the wide range of options for second-year training gives support to the use of the term *PGY2* or *advanced practice residency*, rather than *specialized residency training*, to describe available programs.

A number of the PGY2 options, such as cardiology or oncology, are classic specialty practice areas that would be

By 2011, numerous types of PGY2 residencies were listed on the ASHP accreditation website.

Table 7-1 Options for Accredited PGY2 Residencies*

Ambulatory care

Cardiology pharmacy

Critical care pharmacy

Drug information

Geriatrics pharmacy

Health-system pharmacy administration

Infectious diseases pharmacy

Informatics

Internal medicine pharmacy

Medication-use safety

Nuclear medicine pharmacy

Nutrition support pharmacy

Oncology pharmacy

Pain management and palliative care

Pediatric pharmacy

Pharmacotherapy

Psychiatric pharmacy

Solid organ transplant pharmacy

*There is an option for developing pharmacy residency training in an advanced area of practice (PGY2), although it requires the development of outcomes, goals, and objectives (see the ASHP website for more information about this option and complete titles of other specialty options).
Sources: Adapted from American Society of Health-System Pharmacists. Residency accreditation. http://www.ashp.org/Import/ACCREDITATION/ResidencyAccreditation.aspx. Accessed May 31, 2011; and American College of Clinical Pharmacy. What is a residency and how do I get one? http://www.accp.com/stunet/compass/residency.aspx#pgy-2. Accessed May 31, 2011.

recognized by other healthcare professionals. Other PGY2 residencies, such as ambulatory care or pharmacotherapy, cover much broader areas. Some debate exists within the profession as to whether they are or are not areas of specialty practice. (See Chapter 6, "Ambulatory-Based Residencies," for more discussion.) Some PGY2 options, such as informatics, medication-use safety, or healthcare system pharmacy administration, focus more on healthcare systems than direct patient care activities. Finally, there is a PGY2 option titled Pharmacy Residency Training in an Advanced Area of Practice that provides an option for second-year training in areas other than those listed in Table 7-1. For example, a PGY2 program focusing on emergency medicine could use this option to seek formal accreditation status by developing program outcomes, educational goals and objectives, and a list of important diseases or conditions for guiding residents' training.

Similar to PGY1 residency programs, there are educational outcomes, goals, and objectives for PGY2 programs in the aforementioned areas. These items are individualized for each program, and readers are referred to the residency accreditation webpage for ASHP (http://www.ashp.org/accreditation-residency) for details. Similar to PGY1 programs, second-year programs have required and elective educational outcomes.

For a student or PGY1 resident considering advanced training, there is no shortage of choices for PGY2 areas. For the remainder of this chapter, the term *specialization* will be used interchangeably with PGY2 since all PGY2 programs lead to increased specialization, or advanced practice, to some degree.

SECURING A PGY2 RESIDENCY

• Passion for Area of Advanced Practice or Specialization

Specialization directs a resident down a distinct road in his or her pharmacy career, so a prudent resident should take steps to choose the correct road. There are steps that a prospective advanced practice resident can take to make sure that the advanced practice area is appropriate. First, the candidate should have a definite liking for the area of practice. This may seem obvious, but amazingly, many students and residents consider an area of specialization because they rounded with a great team or had a fantastic preceptor.

> The potential resident should be excited by the actual *area* of specialization.

The potential resident should be excited by the actual *area* of specialization, since he or she will likely have little choice about which other healthcare professionals will share the workplace. The best way a candidate can ensure that he or she has an affinity for the area of specialization is to acquire as much experience in the area as possible (e.g., advanced pharmacy practice experiences as a student, rotations during PGY1 residency). Furthermore, researching the area as much as possible by reading articles, talking to specialists who work in the area, and talking to experienced nonspecialists who might bring a different perspective to the discussion also will be helpful. A prospective advanced practice resident should become familiar with the accreditation standards for PGY2 programs in the area of interest. When considering an area of specialization, the candidate should explore how employment in this area aligns with personal and professional goals. Consequently, potential advanced practice residents should spend time considering their goals and aspirations for their career. In essence, this involves creation of an individualized strategic plan, with a mission, vision, and goals. (See Chapter 18, "Developing a Personal Mission and Leadership Style," for more information). This should be a written plan, although it can and likely will be modified over time. As much as possible, this research into the area should be accomplished prior to PGY2 specialty program application. Neither the potential resident nor the program is well served by scheduling an on-site interview for a candidate who subsequently decides that he or she is not interested in that area.

• Program Fit

After a resident determines that an area of specialization is suitable, the most appropriate program should be identified. The fit should not only be based on objective considerations such as the experience of the program director and key preceptors, but also on less tangible and more subjective feelings that suggest the program will offer a positive experience. **Table 7-2** provides questions to consider when evaluating whether a PGY2 program is a good fit.

Table 7-2 Questions to Consider When Evaluating Whether a PGY2 Program Is a Good Fit for the Applicant

- What is the vision for the pharmacy program and, in particular, the PGY2 residency?

- Is this an established program that has graduated previous specialty residents in the area? If not, does it appear that the necessary infrastructure has been created to make this a quality experience?

- Is the program well structured with an appropriate array of preceptors, rotations, and longitudinal experiences?

- Does the program director, in particular, view the PGY2 residency as a short-term relationship that ends when the resident leaves the program or as a longer-term mutually beneficial relationship?

- What is the experience of the program director and key preceptors?

- How long have the program director and key preceptors been at the site?

- Do all personnel seem content with their positions, and are they enthusiastic about helping to ensure the success of the PGY2 resident and program?

- Do the program director and key preceptors seem to have a desire for ongoing improvement in their clinical and educating skills?

- Do the program director and key preceptors want to practice above the minimum level of competency as exhibited by things such as board certification, participation in scholarly activities, and active membership in professional organizations with presentations at professional meetings?

- Do the program director and key preceptors support the profession through involvement in at least one major pharmacy organization in addition to membership in specialty organizations? (Recognition of the program director by his or her peers in the specialty area could help the resident seek a position following a PGY2 residency.)

> **Table 7-2 Questions to Consider When Evaluating Whether a PGY2 Program Is a Good Fit for the Applicant (*Continued*)**
>
> • Do key administrative personnel, such as the director of pharmacy and/or clinical coordinator, enthusiastically support the PGY2 program?
>
> • Are nonpharmacy personnel supportive of pharmacy and the PGY2 residency?
>
> • Has there been any recent turnover in key personnel at the institution that might affect the specialized program?
>
> • Is education and training part of the mission of the institution?
>
> • Are there any institution-wide changes currently in progress, or expected in the near future, that might affect the PGY2 program in a negative way?
>
> • What types of research have past and/or current residents performed, and were the results presented or published?
>
> • Has the program passed accreditation? If it is a new program, is it seeking accreditation? If the former, what were the noncompliant or partially compliant items? If the latter, does it appear to meet most of the accreditation standards?
>
> Based on the answers to all of these questions and the applicant's impressions, is the program and program director a good fit for the applicant?

For any particular PGY2 specialty, programs may offer a wide range of potential experiences. For example, within critical care, not only are general surgical and medical intensive care units (ICUs) available, but also ICUs based on age (e.g., neonatal, pediatric, and adult) and organ system or type of injury (e.g., burn, cardiac, pulmonary, neurosurgical, trauma). Even within the latter areas, further subspecialization may differentiate critical care residencies, such as an ICU dedicated to the care of patients with strokes. The institution itself may have a specialty focus, such as a cancer center with ICUs that only care for critically ill cancer patients. The variety of experiences available within PGY2 programs should thus be considered, as well as how these experiences align with personal interests and future job possibilities. As wide a net as possible should be cast when initially investigating programs. This approach may take a variety of forms, including discussions with personnel from the programs at professional meetings, residency showcases, or personnel placement services. The program and personnel should be researched via MEDLINE for publications by the program director and key preceptors, as well as face-to-face talks with the program director and any current specialty resident(s) at an event such as the ASHP Midyear Clinical Meeting Residency Showcase. Compared to general program directors, specialists with limited travel funds may choose to attend a meeting in their area of expertise (e.g., attendance at the Society of Critical Care Medicine meeting by critical care pharmacists) rather than more general pharmacy practice meetings. In addition to contacting the program director, applicants may also consider attending meetings related to their PGY2 area of interest in order to meet program directors and other leaders in the field.

Readers are referred to Section II of this book for additional information regarding how to find a residency. There may be some unique aspects related to PGY2 preparation. Some programs require PGY2 applicants to prepare a formal presentation. Residents should inquire about this possibility in advance of the interview. If a presentation is required, determine the appropriate format and topics, length of the presentation, and anticipated audience prior to organizing the material. An on-site interview is also the time to discover the details of the program; the pertinent questions will be similar to those asked by candidates for PGY1 programs. However, in contrast to many general residency programs, many specialty programs have one PGY2 resident per program director, so this relationship is critically important and hopefully lifelong.

Some programs require PGY2 applicants to prepare a formal presentation.

• Early Commitment

The PGY2 residency program director and the PGY1 resident can agree to early commitment and not participate in the match by a process. The early commitment process is appealing for both parties, since they can forgo the uncertainties associated with the match. In fact, some students choose a PGY1 program based on their intended application for a PGY2 program at the same institution. However, for a number of reasons, the early commitment decision should not be taken lightly. The commitment must be made in December when the PGY1 residency is less than half completed. By forgoing the match, the program director may miss a more qualified and compatible applicant, and the PGY1 resident may miss an opportunity to find a PGY2 program that better fits his or her interests and career goals. From a broader perspective, the early commitment process often seems unfair to PGY1 applicants who may be interested in a program but subsequently discover that they do not have an opportunity to interview or apply for the position (see Chapter 16, "The Residency Matching Program," for more information).

The early commitment decision should not be taken lightly.

KEY POINTS

- Before applying for a PGY2 residency, applicants should be sure they have a passion for the PGY2 area of specialization and plan to focus their professional career in that area.

- The applicant should be excited by the area of specialization itself and not just preceptors or allied health professionals who made previous experiences in the area enjoyable.

- Applicants should realize that for any particular PGY2 specialty, programs may offer a wide range of potential experiences, and even within the specialty areas there may be further specialization.

- There is typically one PGY2 resident per program director, so this relationship is critically important for a successful residency and likely forms the basis for a lifelong professional relationship.

- The early commitment process for PGY2 programs has advantages and disadvantages for both the program and the applicant, so the decision to pursue this process requires careful consideration.

REFERENCES

1. American Society of Hospital Pharmacists. ASHP accreditation standard for specialized pharmacy residency training (with guide to interpretation). *Amer J Hosp Pharm*. 1980;37:1229–1232.
2. American Society of Hospital Pharmacists. ASHP supplementary standard and learning objectives for residency training in psychiatric pharmacy practice (supplement to the ASHP accreditation standard for specialized pharmacy residency training). *Amer J Hosp Pharm*. 1980;37:1232–1234.
3. American Society of Hospital Pharmacists. ASHP accreditation standard for specialized pharmacy residency training (with guide to interpretation). *Amer J Hosp Pharm*. 1988;45:1924–1930.
4. American Society of Hospital Pharmacists. ASHP accreditation standard for specialized pharmacy residency training (with guide to interpretation). *Amer J Hosp Pharm*. 1994;51:2034–2041.
5. Teeters JL. New ASHP pharmacy residency accreditation standards. *Amer J Health Syst Pharm*. 2006;63:1012–1018.
6. Daugherty NE, Ryan M, Romanelli F, Smith KM. Board certification of pharmacy residency program directors. *Amer J Health Syst Pharm*. 2010;64:1415–1421.

CHAPTER 8

Nontraditional Pharmacy Residency Programs

Ray R. Maddox and Denise E. Daly

One secret of success in life is for a man to be ready for his opportunity when it comes.

—Benjamin Disraeli

QUESTIONS TO PONDER

1. What is a nontraditional pharmacy residency?
2. Why consider a nontraditional residency?
3. Do nontraditional residents have to give up their current job and pay?
4. Will this kind of residency enhance the career options of a pharmacist?

A nontraditional pharmacy residency is a program designed primarily to accommodate the training needs of pharmacists already in practice. Individuals who select a nontraditional residency complete the residency requirements over two to three years instead of the traditional 12-month residency year.[1-3] Nontraditional residencies are increasing in number to meet the needs of the pharmacy workforce. Whether the nontraditional residency training is stretched over two, three, or more years, the content of the residency program must match the requirements of the American Society of Health-System Pharmacists (ASHP) postgraduate year one (PGY1) standards, provided the program is conducted at a site offering accredited residencies.

> **Individuals who select a nontraditional residency complete the residency requirements over two to three years.**

It is important to remember that not all residency programs, whether traditional or nontraditional, are accredited.

Nontraditional residency programs have been developed in response to unmet needs of both the profession and the practitioner. The vision for the future is that completion of an accredited residency program will be essential for a pharmacist to achieve his or her full potential in improving medication therapy outcomes in all practice settings.[4] In order for the profession to provide residency training for both new graduates and current practitioners, significant growth in the number of available residency programs will need to occur. Nontraditional residencies can help fill the gap by providing opportunities for current practitioners who initially chose not to complete a residency or were unable to commit to a traditional residency.

STRUCTURE AND TRAINING CONTENT

Requirements for residency content and rotations can be found in the ASHP accreditation standards for PGY1 programs (see Chapter 3, "Postgraduate Year One (PGY1) Pharmacy Residency Programs").[5-7] The primary differences between traditional and nontraditional residencies are the length of time required to complete the residency and the type of individual enrolled. Traditional residents are usually new graduates completing a one-year experience, whereas nontraditional residents continue to fulfill staff pharmacist responsibilities during their residency. Therefore, training rotations for nontraditional residents are scheduled around and in conjunction with their staffing responsibilities. Some residency training activities are longitudinal, meaning they occur over the length of the residency versus being completed in a fixed time, such as a four-week rotation. These activities include attendance at various committee meetings, conducting medication use evaluations, completing a research project, and writing reports and/or manuscripts. Nontraditional residents may be required to participate in some of these functions during the time they are assigned to pharmacist staffing responsibilities.

> **Nontraditional residents continue to fulfill staff pharmacist responsibilities during their residency.**

All residency programs should be tailored to the needs of the individual resident. Given that nontraditional residents will be engaged in clinical practice before beginning the residency, specific content of the nontraditional residency should be built upon the competencies already possessed by the individual. Nontraditional residents must challenge themselves to go beyond the duties they usually undertake on a day-to-day basis as an employee. Nontraditional residents can be expected to participate in more complex patient care cases, complete greater in-depth research projects, assume broader leadership roles, and expand the overall scope of their pharmacy practice.

The nontraditional resident will spend a total of 12 months involved in residency activities, but the residency months will not be consecutive. Nontraditional programs schedule their residency months based on the needs of the institution, as well as those of the resident. In some programs, a nontraditional resident may spend one of every three months in residency activities, and other programs may schedule two consecutive months out of every six months as residency months.[1]

ADMISSION REQUIREMENTS AND ACCREDITATION

Individuals admitted to nontraditional residencies must meet the same qualifications outlined in the ASHP standards for all resident applicants. Admission into a nontraditional program may require that the nontraditional candidate be a current employee of the institution offering the program. This approach limits the pool of applicants but ensures that the individual is committed to the institution and has already demonstrated his or her qualifications as a candidate. ASHP accreditation standards thus do not differ between traditional and nontraditional programs. The nontraditional program simply represents an alternative scheduling process compared with the 12-month traditional schedule.

> Individuals admitted to nontraditional residencies must meet the same qualifications outlined in the ASHP standards for all resident applicants.

NONTRADITIONAL RESIDENCY CONSIDERATIONS

Nontraditional residencies are ideal for *practicing* pharmacists who are already functioning in the workforce. As nonresidency-trained clinical pharmacists mature in their practice, they may find that their career goals have changed. They may be motivated to take on a more active direct patient care role and expanded clinical duties but feel they lack the training and direction to do so. Nontraditional residency programs are uniquely situated to bridge the gap for pharmacists who find themselves in this position. A nontraditional program can provide the avenue for currently practicing pharmacists to pursue the advanced training they require to expand their practice capabilities. In these instances, the programs are geared toward recruiting pharmacists already in practice who are seeking to broaden their careers. Nontraditional residency programs also may be used as a recruiting tool to entice new graduates.

> A nontraditional program can provide the avenue for currently practicing pharmacists to pursue the advanced training they require to expand their practice capabilities.

Upon employment, the new graduate would simultaneously assume the role of a newly hired pharmacist and a nontraditional resident. The newly hired resident gains work experience and the benefits of completing a residency, and the institution gains a multiple-year commitment from a pharmacist in advanced training. Evidence suggests that pharmacists who have completed postgraduate residency or fellowship training are more satisfied with their careers than those who have not completed this type of training.[8]

As previously noted, nontraditional residencies are intended for pharmacists who are in practice and who are completing their residency on a part-time basis. Individual institutions that offer nontraditional residencies will likely structure the pay and benefits for nontraditional residents differently. For instance, some programs may pay the nontraditional resident a full pharmacist wage during resident and staffing months,[1] and others adjust the pay downward during residency rotation months.[2,3] Although a nontraditional resident is not guaranteed a higher-paying position after the residency is complete, the graduate can expect continued employment at the institution.

Pharmacy practice, particularly in hospitals and healthcare systems, has become dependent on well-trained clinical practitioners. Although doctor of pharmacy education programs produce graduates with the fundamental tools required for licensure, the complexity in hospital pharmacotherapy management often necessitates advanced knowledge and training. Additionally, pharmacy organizations are increasing their advocacy for residency training for all healthcare system pharmacists.[4] Pharmacists who lack residency training and are employed in hospitals and healthcare systems may be at a disadvantage in the provision of many clinical services. Career advancement also may be negatively affected. Therefore, healthcare system pharmacists should strongly consider taking advantage of nontraditional residency programs when this option is available.

> Healthcare system pharmacists should strongly consider taking advantage of nontraditional residency programs when this option is available.

Pharmacists interested in pursuing a nontraditional residency should research the benefits of residency-level education and ascertain how residency training would benefit their personal and professional development. Residency training can also contribute to reenergizing seasoned practitioners who have become comfortable in the requirements of their day-to-day routine. When choosing nontraditional residency training, pharmacists should thoroughly evaluate a program's offerings just as they would for a traditional residency program. For instance, potential nontraditional residents should evaluate whether the program is ASHP accredited, how long the PGY1 program has existed, the variety of clinical and nonclinical rotations, and if there are enough residency preceptors with sufficient depths of experience to enhance the nontraditional applicant's existing practice credentials. Additionally, individuals interested in nontraditional residencies should perform a thorough self-assessment of their career goals, strengths, and weaknesses.

BENEFITS AND LIMITATIONS OF NONTRADITIONAL RESIDENCIES

• Benefits

Nontraditional residencies offer several benefits to the pharmacist who is already in the workforce, as well as to the sites.

BENEFITS FOR THE PHARMACIST

- Completion of advanced residency training without having to forfeit a job and relocate

- Maintenance of a sustainable income during the residency training experience

- Continuation of family stability because of no separation during the term of the residency

- Achievement of career-enhancing training and skills from a structured advanced-practice experience

- Attainment of an additional credential: the certificate of residency training

BENEFITS FOR THE SITE

- Provides a recruitment incentive for selected employees

- Creates an internal process for career enhancement and advancement

- Retains employees

- Strengthens the internal workforce for expansion of clinical services

• Limitations

As with all life experiences, the nontraditional approach to residency training may possess some inherent limitations. Among these possible limitations are the following:

- The amount of income may be less than that of a full-time pharmacist.

- Two or more years are required to complete the residency.

- The intermittent process of completing the residency may interfere with the continuity of completing various residency projects and longitudinal training activities.

- Time management for the resident during the residency may be challenging since most nontraditional residents will have multiple personal, nonprofessional life commitments they must also manage.

- Scheduling and coordination of work schedules, residency rotations, and personal time may be difficult.

Nontraditional pharmacy residents are typically highly motivated individuals who have concluded that advanced-level skills are essential to achieve their professional goals and objectives. These individuals are willing to make sacrifices to

Nontraditional pharmacy residents are typically highly motivated individuals who have concluded that advanced-level skills are essential.

achieve these professional goals by giving up personal time, comfort, and sometimes income for the short term. They generally demonstrate leadership qualities and a high measure of professionalism in their practice prior to entering the residency. Individuals who display these characteristics and want to advance their practice should consider an opportunity to complete a nontraditional residency if it arises.

KEY POINTS

- Nontraditional pharmacy residencies are a viable and important alternative for advanced practice training of pharmacists who are already in the workforce.

- These residencies are growing in number, particularly in facilities where traditional residencies are in place.

- Nontraditional residencies offer similar content as traditional residencies over a longer time period.

- These residencies enhance the growth of clinical practitioners already practicing within the profession.

REFERENCES

1. Winegardner ML, Davis SL, Szandzik EG, Kalus JS. Nontraditional pharmacy residency at a large teaching hospital. *Am J Health Syst Pharm.* 2010;67:366–370.
2. Johns Hopkins Medicine Department of Pharmacy. Non-traditional flex PGY1 pharmacy residency program. http://www.hopkinsmedicine.org/pharmacy/residents/programs/Non-traditionalFlex_PGY1.html. Accessed March 31, 2011.
3. Kern Medical Center. Pharmacy practice residency program. http://www.kernmedicalcenter.com/body.cfm?id=384. Accessed March 31, 2011.
4. Teeters JL, Brueckl M, Burns A, Flynn A, Webb E. Pharmacy residency training in the future: a stakeholders' roundtable discussion. *Am J Health Syst Pharm.* 2005;62:1817–1820.
5. American Society of Health-System Pharmacists. ASHP regulations on accreditation of pharmacy residencies. http://www.ashp.org/s_ashp/docs/files/RTP_ResidencyAccredRegulation.pdf. Accessed March 31, 2011.
6. American Society of Health-System Pharmacists. ASHP accreditation standard for postgraduate year one (PGY1) pharmacy residency programs. http://www.ashp.org/s_ashp/docs/files/RTP_PGY1AccredStandard.pdf. Accessed March 31, 2011.
7. American Society of Health-System Pharmacists. ASHP accreditation standard for postgraduate year two (PGY2) pharmacy residency programs. http://www.ashp.org/s_ashp/docs/files/RTP_PGY2AccredStandard.pdf. Accessed March 31, 2011.
8. Padiyara RS, Komperda KE. Effect of postgraduate training on job and career satisfaction among health-system pharmacists. *Am J Health Syst Pharm.* 2010;67:1093–1100.

Finding the Right Residency

Anna M. Wodlinger Jackson, Section Editor

■ Checklist: Securing a Pharmacy Residency

Complete this checklist to ensure adequate preparation and application for a residency. (Note: The acronyms are defined at the end of the checklist.)

Throughout Pharmacy School (Start Early)

❑ Contemplate your career options and related residency requirements.

❑ Get involved and develop your leadership skills (e.g., organizations, extracurricular activities).

❑ Begin to network; get to know your faculty members and those in the pharmacy community.

❑ Obtain intern hours at a practice site that is consistent with your career goals, when known.

❑ Consider research opportunities (e.g., elective courses, work studies).

❑ Enroll in distinctive didactic electives oriented toward patient care.

❑ Develop and revise your curriculum vitae with input from others (faculty, friends, family).

❑ Consider developing a residency applicant portfolio.

❑ Compete in a local and potentially national competition:
  - ASHP Clinical Skills Competition
  - ACCP Clinical Pharmacy Challenge
  - APhA–ASP Patient Counseling Competition
  - NCPA Pruitt-Schutte Business Plan Competition

❑ Choose challenging APPEs with high-level, direct patient care activities.

❑ Attend the ASHP MCM (held annually in December) as an observer, if feasible.

❑ Attend local or regional residency showcases, where applicable.

Final Professional Year

August	❑ Construct a personal inventory (e.g., career goals, strengths, areas to improve). ❑ Plan travel to the ASHP MCM. ❑ Determine if you will use the ASHP Personnel Placement Service (not required)
September	❑ For guidance, seek out previous graduates who enrolled in residency programs.
October	❑ Revise your curriculum vitae with input from others (faculty, friends, family). ❑ Finalize your residency applicant portfolio, if developed. ❑ Attend local or regional residency showcases, where applicable.
November	❑ Search the ASHP database for residencies that match your career interests. ❑ Develop a list of programs to consider at the MCM Residency Showcase. ❑ Request faculty and preceptors to serve as references. ❑ Collect and begin working on applications.
December	❑ Provide references with necessary information early (e.g., materials, deadlines). ❑ Attend the ASHP MCM (schedule travel early). ❑ Attend the ASHP MCM Residency Showcase (map out each day in advance). ❑ Attend the ASHP Personnel Placement Service (if chosen to use) ❑ Send thank-you notes to midyear interviewers and references. ❑ Sign up for the match via NMS (the deadline is usually mid-January). ❑ Submit program applications (due mid-December to early January).
January-February	❑ Sign up for the match via NMS (if not already completed). ❑ Interview with programs, where interviews are offered

March	❑ Submit your rank order list to NMS (see website for exact date).
	❑ Match results are announced (see website for exact date).
	❑ Scramble if unmatched (address immediately when unfilled list is provided).
April-June	❑ Obtain pharmacy licensure promptly.
	❑ Check with residency program regarding unique requirements (e.g., credentialing).
July	❑ Start residency program.

■ Key Websites Related to Finding the Right Residency

(Note: The acronyms are defined at the end of the list.)

ASHP Residency Directory: www.ashp.org/ResidencyDirectory

ASHP Residency Accreditation: http://www.ashp.org/accreditation

ACCP Directory of Residencies, Fellowships, and Graduate Programs: www.accp.com/resandfel/index.aspx

APhA Community Pharmacy Residencies: http://www.pharmacist.com/residencies

AMCP Residency Opportunities: http://www.amcp.org/residencies

National Matching Services: www.natmatch.com/ashprmp

Acronyms

ACCP: American College of Clinical Pharmacy
AMCP: Academy of Managed Care Pharmacy
APhA: American Pharmacists Association
APPE: Advanced Pharmacy Practice Experience
ASHP: American Society of Health-System Pharmacists
ASP: Academy of Student Pharmacists
MCM: Midyear Clinical Meeting
NCPA: National Community Pharmacists Association
NMS: National Matching Services

CHAPTER 9

The Curriculum Vitae and Letter of Intent

Jason C. Gallagher

If you call failures experiments, you can put them in your resume and claim them as achievements.

—**Mason Cooley**

QUESTIONS TO PONDER

1. How should one compose a letter of intent?

2. What are the typical components of one's curriculum vitae (CV)?

3. How can the CV most optimally highlight a residency applicant's qualifications and make him or her stand out?

4. How does the CV evolve throughout one's career?

5. What are common errors when composing a CV?

Nearly all students are familiar with the term *curriculum vitae*, though they may be less comfortable with the process of writing one and differentiating it from resumes prepared for past jobs. Resumes are not appropriate for residency candidates. The lack of fixed rules about CV writing can make the venture frustrating for students and young practitioners who are writing one for the first time. For residency applicants, concurrent with the submission of a CV is a letter of intent. A letter of intent acts as a notification of an individual's application for a residency or employment. It is an excellent

Resumes are not appropriate for residency candidates.

opportunity to highlight the virtues of one's CV and to fill in any gaps that may appear on a CV due to life circumstances.

The term *curriculum vitae* literally means "course of one's life." The CV has come to be a record of one's relevant professional history and accomplishments presented in a concise, readable format. This differs from a resume, which is a skill-based, extremely concise one- or two-page document written to obtain a particular position. The CV is more thorough and contains a complete record of one's experiences, not just a listing of skills and previous employers. The potential employer should be able to review a CV quickly to ascertain a candidate's work experience and educational background. The CV of a pharmacy residency candidate includes elements such as advanced pharmacy practice experiences completed, project experience, publications and presentations, extracurricular activities, and other pertinent facts.[1]

> The potential employer should be able to review a CV quickly to ascertain a candidate's work experience and educational background.

GENERAL FORMATTING FOR CURRICULUM VITAE AND LETTERS OF INTENT

In general, the CV and letter of intent are printed on one side of good quality white (or near white) 8.5" × 11" paper. The layout should be highly organized with ample white space, justified to the left margin, and with 1-inch margins on all sides. The text font should be consistent, with preference oftentimes given to a sans serif font (e.g., Arial, Tahoma, Verdana). The fonts are generally 10–12 points and should never be less than 10 points. The formatting should be consistent throughout the documents.

For CVs, use boldface, capital letters, or underline to make category headings stand out, as appropriate. In addition, a varied design format (e.g., bullets, lines, shading) can be used to define transitions between sections. Information should be presented in a consistent format, either in chronological or reverse chronological order; the latter is most common and logical for residency candidates' CVs.

> If the applicant anticipates sending documents via e-mail, consider saving the document as a PDF file.

If the applicant anticipates sending documents via e-mail, consider saving the document as a PDF file, which keeps the formatting consistent among computers. It is important to exclude information from CVs regarding physical characteristics and other personal information, such as age, gender, ethnicity, marital status, and political and religious affiliations.

LETTER OF INTENT STRUCTURE

The structure of the letter of intent will vary based on the individual and the residency program to which the candidate is applying. The candidate should follow the application guidelines closely to ensure the letter includes all the required elements. Some programs have specific information that must be included in the letter. Although there will be common items that can be cut and pasted from one letter of intent to another, each letter should be unique.

It is important for the applicant to write the letter in a professional way that follows a business letter format. The letter should be written in first person, but most people argue that the initial paragraph should not begin with "I." By following a standard format, residency programs can consider the applicant quickly along with the probable high number of other applications. **Appendix A** of this chapter provides an example letter of intent.

• Detailed Elements

The letter of intent starts with an introductory paragraph. This short section expresses the applicant's interest in the program, which should identify the organization directly. The paragraph may also contain comments regarding how the applicant learned about the residency program, particularly if it is through a personal connection to the program, such as a former resident or a discussion with a program representative at a meeting. This paragraph may also highlight aspects about the program that are particularly attractive to the candidate—the more specific, the better.

The next section highlights abilities and why the applicant should be chosen for an interview. The goal is to show why the applicant is a valuable candidate the program should choose for an on-site interview. This section will vary greatly from one applicant to the next and may contain more than one paragraph. It is important to highlight any evidence that the applicant has leadership qualities, as well as any experiences that make the applicant stand out from others. The applicant should word this section to emphasize key attributes and abilities. Overt bragging is a negative, though the letter of intent is not a time to be humble, either. If any apparent gaps exist in an applicant's CV or transcript, such as taking a year off from pharmacy school to attend to an ailing family member, it is important to explain the gaps here.

The final paragraph of the letter provides a conclusion. This short ending reiterates the specific name of the program and, at a minimum, expresses the applicant's level of interest. This paragraph may also restate how the residency program could benefit from the applicant.

CURRICULUM VITAE STRUCTURE

CVs differ greatly in their structure from person to person, and particularly from profession to profession. CVs for pharmacists should contain certain common elements. The applicant's full legal name or first name, middle initial, and last name along with contact information should be prominent on the top of a CV, including permanent and current addresses and a professional e-mail address. Consider including phone numbers for day and evening and a fax number, if applicable. Headers or footers may include the name, date, page number (e.g., Page 2 of 6), and "Curriculum Vitae," which are helpful if pages get misplaced or out of order.

The sections that follow are supplemented by an example residency applicant's CV, as shown in **Appendix B** of this chapter.

• Detailed Elements

Listing a professional goal or objective is optional; if it is included, it should not be too vague or too specific. If the candidate is seeking a particular residency, the objective should be consistent with the position.

Educational experiences should include courses of study in all institutions attended, including prepharmacy work. Grade point averages (GPAs) may be included if greater than 3.0, but it is best to exclude them if the GPA from one course of study (e.g., prepharmacy curriculum) is greater than 3.0 but another (e.g., pharmacy school) is not. The level of academic distinction (e.g., magna cum laude) also may be included, as applicable. Be sure to correctly spell the name of each institution and signify degrees. Pharmacy schools in the United States award the *doctor of pharmacy* degree, not a *pharmacy doctorate* or *doctorate of pharmacy*.

> Pharmacy schools in the United States award the *doctor of pharmacy* degree.

Licensure and certifications can be listed early in the CV. However, this section may need to be minimized if the residency applicant has few or no items to list. For those seeking a postgraduate year one (PGY1) residency, certificates and registered internships should be listed. Postgraduate year two (PGY2) residents should also list pharmacy licenses.

Work and professional experiences should contain a listing of jobs or internships previously and currently held. Some candidates also include bullet points about each position to describe the activities performed. If this is done, then several rules should be followed. First, a general rule of outlining is to include at least two points per position. Additionally, ensure that the tense of each position and task is correct (e.g., one does not "dispense" medication at a job that is no longer held). Nonpharmacy positions may be included, particularly for candidates with significant experience before attending pharmacy school. Ensure that there are no unexplained gaps in the work experience. Although education easily explains a lack of employment, a gap between jobs without concurrent schooling may look questionable to a potential employer. If such a gap exists, consider explaining it up front in the letter of intent.

A listing of pharmacy practice experiences (introductory and advanced) is a given in a student pharmacist's CV, but the elements to include when listing them can be confusing. Include all completed and pending experiences (if they have been scheduled) on the CV, and for each one include the preceptor's correctly spelled name and credentials, site of the experience, and dates they were completed. Preceptor listings are more important than they may seem. These listings may serve as a conversation point during an interview or provide a personal connection between the applicant and the interviewer.

Other sections that may be listed at this point in the CV depend on the achievements of the applicant. Honors and awards should be listed prominently in the CV if there are notable achievements. The same holds true for research experience, publications, and abstracts or posters.

Research experience is attractive to many residency programs, since the completion of a major project is an expectation of a residency. All research experience should be listed, from both pharmacy school and any undergraduate or other experience. Be sure to include the correctly spelled name of any advisors. Overall, research experience is a significant positive. However, be aware that residency programs are clinical programs, and they may question if a student with a very high degree of basic science research experience is well suited for a clinical training program. This can be explained in the letter of intent or during an interview.

Overall, research experience is a significant positive.

Publications are an obvious plus on any CV, especially for a young practitioner or student. Publications submitted for publication or in press (submitted and accepted) also may be listed. Most students will not have published anything at the time of the residency application process, and residency programs do not expect publications; however, articles in publications such as journals of local pharmacy associations, hospital newsletters, newspapers, and other nonscientific journals are worth listing. The formatting should follow the guidelines for biomedical journals. Check style guides such as *The Chicago Manual of Style* or the *AMA Manual of Style*. If the applicant has an abstract and/or poster, that can be listed separately.

The presentations area of a CV is one that can grow quite a bit while a student completes his or her educational program. Student pharmacists who are preparing a CV for the first time often wonder what counts as a presentation. Each presentation completed inside of the classroom and on advanced pharmacy practice experiences should be listed. This includes common presentations on rotations, such as journal clubs and case presentations. Never assume that the reader knows that students

Never assume that the reader knows that students complete case presentations on rotations.

complete case presentations on rotations. Presentation on a CV may catch an interviewer's interest and spark a conversation about that topic that can help a candidate stand out. Some students include listings of journal club and case presentations, nursing in-services, and presentations to the medical team under the pharmacy practice experiences heading, but it is better to put them in a section of their own where they can stand out and are easier to read. In addition to the presentations that take place on rotations and in classes, any poster presentations at national, regional, or local meetings should be on the CV as well. Given the variety in types of presentations, it is important to include the type of presentation and audience to whom the presentation was given (e.g., lecture given to pharmacy faculty and students in Acute Care Elective (DPET 802), seminar given to pharmacy faculty and staff, in-service given to nursing and medical staff). A separate section of abstracts and posters is not a requirement, but it is an option that helps highlight a candidate's more unique work.

Memberships in professional organizations, committees, and community activities should always be on a student's CV, either together or separately. Related to these items, leadership roles and positions on organizational committees should be highlighted. Many residency programs look specifically for evidence of leadership on candidates' CVs, and extracurricular and professional organizations are good documentation. As with professional experience, this section may be an area where bulleted lists allow for elaboration on activities performed for a specific organization.

Finally, additional sections that some individuals may include are teaching experience and volunteer work outside of extracurricular activities. For teaching experience, list the job title (instructor, lecturer, teaching assistant) followed by the course title, including the course number. The affiliated institution should be included along with the date or date range during which the instruction was provided. Clinical and laboratory instruction also should be included.

• Translating Achievements into the Curriculum Vitae

When composing a CV, it can be helpful to remember its purpose: to chronicle one's professional experiences and work. As such, it is important to be thorough, not humble, when listing achievements. Never assume that an interviewer is familiar with the applicant's academic program; even alumni of pharmacy schools cannot follow curricular changes. If something seems like a noteworthy accomplishment, it is, and it should be listed in the CV. Remembering past achievements, presentations, and positions can be challenging, so it is best to keep a CV current with each accomplishment as it is completed to avoid suffering from a lack of recall later. For all items listed on the CV, maintaining a folder of handouts, slides, and other related materials is helpful when it comes time to prepare for an interview (see Chapter 10, "The Residency Applicant's Portfolio," and Chapter 14, "The Onsite Interview").

• Is That Enough?

Again, there are no fixed rules for how big a CV should be or even what content it should include. A CV grows as one's career progresses, and the relatively short CV of a student pharmacist midway through a professional program will become much longer after a year of advanced pharmacy practice experiences. Although it is important to be thorough in constructing a CV, the content must be legitimate. Experienced interviewers can easily identify a CV that is being stretched with obvious fluff. Anything listed on the CV is fair game during an interview, so be prepared to discuss any listed topic.

THE CURRICULUM VITAE AS A LIVING AND CHANGING DOCUMENT

As a record of professional accomplishments, the CV changes over time. Eventually, as one progresses from student to resident to clinician, the magnitude of accomplishments generally increases, and the content of the CV should follow. Student CVs often contain more detail about lower-level presentations, advanced pharmacy practice experiences, and course work compared to CVs of more experienced practitioners. There is nothing wrong with that, and the more content on a CV that can catch a reviewer's eye, the better. Pharmacy residents rotate through many clinical areas, complete multiple advanced pharmacy practice experiences, and design and implement clinical research projects. All of these areas should be included on a CV as they are achieved. The CVs of more experienced practitioners usually lack areas like rotations completed and in-house presentations like journal clubs; these are eventually replaced by poster and platform presentations at local or national meetings.

• Dos and Don'ts

Although each person's CV is unique and few true rules exist for CV writing, there are a few things to avoid. Keep in mind that the CV is meant to be easily read, and any CV that confuses the reader has failed in its purpose of conveying experience clearly. A summary of common dos and don'ts is listed in **Table 9-1**.

Table 9-1 Dos and Don'ts in CV Preparation

Do	Don't
Keep the CV professional from start to finish.	Include spelling or grammatical errors.
Include current contact information, including a professional e-mail address.	List a casual-sounding e-mail addresses (e.g., "cheerfan23@email.com") or have an unprofessional voice mail greeting.
List the entire CV in either chronological or reverse chronological order.	Shift the order of the CV from section to section.
Use the correct tense when describing current and past positions.	Include personal information that would not be appropriate for interview discussion.
Spell all names correctly on the CV with correct degrees and other credentials.	Use a large font and wide margins to make the CV appear longer than it is.
List the degree or anticipated degree correctly.	Use CV or resume templates in word processing programs.

• Bragging Versus Explaining

Someone reading a CV should quickly become familiar with the writer's body of professional work and accomplishments. Those accomplishments need to be listed in order to impress, but they should not be listed in a way that is disproportional to actual roles on projects or positions in organizations. For example, student pharmacists or residents who were lab technicians on funded studies should not list a $1.5 million grant on their CV, but rather they should simply describe the activities performed as a study coinvestigator or coordinator. Additionally, wording group projects as solitary accomplishments can backfire if the CV reader is familiar with the other members of a group. Be complete, but be honest.

• Personal Versus Professional

The CV is a listing of professional work, not one's personal life. Omit any content from the CV that could be seen as controversial. If an e-mail address can link someone to a page of photos from spring break, it is best to use another one (e.g., Gmail account).

STANDOUT FEATURES OF EXCELLENT CURRICULUM VITAE

Neatness, professionalism, and appropriate content make a CV stand out from those in a crowd of similarly accomplished people. Nothing substitutes for content; however, more accomplished candidates may have an apparent advantage, but CVs that hide those accomplishments in poor organization, grammatical errors, or a lack of clarity are significant detractors. Ensure that there are *absolutely* no spelling errors on the CV. Proofread the CV several times and have it reviewed by a third party. It also may be helpful to have someone with no medical background review the CV to provide a different perspective.

> Ensure that there are *absolutely* no spelling errors on the CV.

Students should not be intimidated by the more lengthy CVs of residents they work with or other more experienced practitioners. Everybody starts somewhere, and in time, the CV naturally grows.

KEY POINTS

- A letter of intent acts as both a notification of an individual's application for a residency and an opportunity to highlight individual strengths.

- The CV has numerous standard components along with several areas that are optional based on the background of the applicant.

- The CV should be clear, thorough, honest, and professional; it also should be highly organized, devoid of spelling and grammatical errors, and easy to read.

- The CV should highlight positions of leadership and involvement in organizations outside the classroom; many residency programs actively look for evidence of leadership skills.

- Anything listed on a CV is fair game during an interview.

REFERENCES

1. Gallagher JC, Wodlinger Jackson AM. How to write a curriculum vitae. *Am J Health Syst Pharm.* 2010;67:446–447.

APPENDIX A
Example Letter of Intent

December 19, 20XX

Jason C. Gallagher, PharmD, BCPS
Director, Pharmacy Practice Residency
Temple University Hospital
Department of Pharmacy Services
3401 North Broad Street
Philadelphia, Pennsylvania 19140
jason.gallagher@temple.edu

Dear Dr. Gallagher:

It is with great enthusiasm that I submit this letter of intent for the postgraduate year one (PGY1) pharmacy residency at Temple University Hospital. I learned of this program from one of my mentors, Dr. John Smith, and he spoke very highly of the program. Since learning about the residency, my interactions with the program leadership and current residents demonstrate this residency is exactly what I seek in postgraduate training.

The enclosed application materials and curriculum vitae provide an overview of my training and experience. I am a motivated, hardworking student who would excel during your residency. In May, I will graduate from the Bill Gatton College of Pharmacy, East Tennessee State University (ETSU). During my time at ETSU, I have been active both on local and statewide levels. Additionally, I have chosen to take on unique opportunities to grow and develop as a student pharmacist, including certificates, research opportunities, distinctive electives, and a publication. For one of my didactic electives, I enrolled in Pharmacy Practice Research/Scholarship. This experience gave me firsthand knowledge regarding research, and I was fortunate to present the study findings as a poster at the American College of Clinical Pharmacy Annual Meeting. I have also endeavored to complete challenging advanced pharmacy practice experiences (APPEs), including an extra APPE beyond program requirements. Overall, ETSU is a challenging Doctor of Pharmacy program that has developed my critical problem-solving skills.

The residency program at Temple University Hospital distinctively meets my professional goals. I am a goal-oriented individual that would excel in the program. I hope the residency selection committee looks favorably on my application.

Sincerely,

John J. Doe, BSc, Doctor of Pharmacy Candidate
Bill Gatton College of Pharmacy
East Tennessee State University

APPENDIX B
Example Curriculum Vitae

Curriculum Vitae

John J. Doe, BSc, Doctor of Pharmacy Candidate
114 Anywhere Avenue
Johnson City, Tennessee 37614
johnjdoe@gmail.com
555-867-5309

December 20XX

Professional Goal

To secure a postgraduate year one (PGY1) residency and excel as a pharmacist who provides direct patient care in a hospital setting.

Education

Doctor of Pharmacy   Expected, May 20XX
Bill Gatton College of Pharmacy
East Tennessee State University
Johnson City, Tennessee
Current GPA 3.7

Bachelor of Science in Chemistry   20XX–20XX
Duke University
Durham, North Carolina
GPA 3.6

Licensure and Certifications

Advanced cardiac life support (ACLS)   20XX–present

Pharmacy-based immunization delivery   20XX–present
certificate (APhA)

Pharmaceutical care for patients with   20XX–present
diabetes certificate (APhA)

Basic life support (BLS)   20XX–present

Work and Professional Experience

Pharmacy Practice Intern   20XX–present
East Tennessee State University
Medical Center
Johnston City, Tennessee

Pharmacy Practice Intern   20XX–20XX
Crouch's Ideal Drug Store
Asheville, North Carolina

Pharmacy Practice Experiences

Advanced

Infectious Diseases Elective, APPE 7028   Expected, April 20XX
Temple University Health System
Jason C. Gallagher, PharmD, BCPS
(AQ Infectious Diseases)

Cardiology Elective, APPE 7039   Expected, March 20XX
University of North Carolina Hospitals
Jo Ellen Rodgers, PharmD, FCCP, BCPS
(AQ Cardiology)

Critical Care Elective, APPE 7019   Expected, February 20XX
University of Arizona Medical Center
Brian L. Erstad, PharmD, FASHP,
FCCM, FCCP

Pediatrics Elective, APPE 7024   Expected, January 20XX
Medical University of South Carolina
Children's Hospital
Dominic P. Ragucci, PharmD, BCPS

Oncology Elective, APPE 7034   November 20XX
East Tennessee State University
Medical Center
John B. Bossaer, PharmD, BCPS

Acute Care Practice II, APPE 6503   October 20XX
East Tennessee State University
Medical Center
Freddy M. Creekmore, PharmD, BCPS

Ambulatory Care Practice I, APPE 6004   September 20XX
East Tennessee State University
Family Physicians
L. Brian Cross, PharmD, CDE

Acute Care Practice I, APPE 6003   August 20XX
East Tennessee State University
Medical Center
David W. Stewart, PharmD, BCPS

Community Practice, APPE 6002   July 20XX
Ukrop's Pharmacy
Jean-Venable Goode, PharmD, BCPS,
FAPhA, FCCP

Institutional Practice, APPE 6001   June 20XX
University of North Carolina Hospitals
Stephen F. Eckel, PharmD, MHA, BCPS,
FAPhA, FASHP

Introductory

Clinical (third year), PMPR 4341   20XX–20XX
East Tennessee State University
Medical Center
Johnson City, Tennessee

Institutional Practice (second year), PMPR 4332   Summer 20XX
East Tennessee State University
Medical Center
Johnson City, Tennessee

Community Practice (second year), PMPR 4322   Summer 20XX
Bob's Pharmacy
Johnson City, Tennessee

Institutional Practice (first year), PMPR 3141   Spring 20XX
East Tennessee State University
Medical Center
Johnson City, Tennessee

Community Practice (first year), PMPR 3141   Fall 20XX
SVC Pharmacy
Johnson City, Tennessee

Honors and Awards

Rho Chi Honor Society, Bill Gatton College of Pharmacy (ETSU), 20XX

Dean's List (all semesters), Bill Gatton College of Pharmacy (ETSU), 20XX

Phi Lambda Sigma Pharmacy Leadership Society, Bill Gatton College of Pharmacy (ETSU), 20XX

Regent (President), Epsilon Zeta Chapter of Kappa Psi, Bill Gatton College of Pharmacy (ETSU), 20XX

Class President (first year), Bill Gatton College of Pharmacy (ETSU), 20XX

Research Experience

Doe JJ, Crouch MA. A cost-effectiveness analysis of anticoagulation strategies in atrial fibrillation; 20XX–20XX.

Publications

Doe JJ. New guidelines from US, international societies. *Cardiovasc Pharmacother Q Rep*. 20XX;3:4.

Abstracts and Posters

Doe JJ, Crouch MA. A cost-effectiveness analysis of anticoagulation strategies in atrial fibrillation. Abstract presented at: 20XX ACCP Annual Meeting: October XX–XX, 20XX; Nashville, Tennessee.

Presentations

Doe JJ. Statins for the acute treatment of aneurismal subarachnoid hemorrhage. Clinical Seminar II (PMPR 5461). Johnson City, Tennessee. Expected January X, 20XX.

Doe JJ. Drug-drug interactions with new oncology agents. In-service provided to healthcare professionals in oncology. November X, 20XX.

Doe JJ. Steroid use in patients with chronic obstructive pulmonary disease: a critical appraisal. In-service provided to healthcare professionals in adult medicine. October X, 20XX.

Doe JJ. An update of the American Diabetes Association (ADA) guidelines. In-service provided to healthcare professionals in the ambulatory care clinic. September X, 20XX.

Doe JJ. New anticoagulant strategies in atrial fibrillation. In-service provided to acute care team. August X, 20XX.

Memberships

Tennessee Pharmacists Association	20XX–present
Rho Chi Honor Society	20XX–present
Phi Lambda Sigma Pharmacy Leadership Society	20XX–present
American College of Clinical Pharmacy (ACCP)	20XX–present
American Society of Health-System Pharmacists (ASHP)	20XX–present
Kappa Psi Pharmaceutical Fraternity	20XX–present

Committees

Dean's Students Advisory Council (DSAC)	20XX–20XX

Community Activities

Johnson City Downtown Clinic Johnson City, Tennessee	20XX–present
Remote Area Medical (RAM) Bristol Motor Speedway Bristol, Tennessee	April 20XX

CHAPTER 10

The Residency Applicant's Portfolio

Jo Ellen Rodgers

The process of creating [a portfolio] is generally much more important and meaningful than the end product.

—**Ohio State University Center for the Advancement of Teaching**

QUESTIONS TO PONDER

1. What is a portfolio, and how does it relate to one's curriculum vitae (CV)?

2. When should a residency applicant start developing a portfolio?

3. Should all residency applicants develop a portfolio?

4. How should the portfolio be used by the residency applicant after it has been developed?

The development of a residency applicant's portfolio is still a relatively new concept. The term *portfolio* has different meanings depending on the situation. In short, the residency applicant's portfolio is used to display in more detail key items listed in one's CV, and it is primarily used during interviews. The process of developing a portfolio is important on its own. The purpose of this chapter is to give a brief history of portfolios, describe the typical content of a residency applicant's portfolio, and review how the portfolio can be used by the applicant after it is developed.

BRIEF HISTORY

In the education field, the use of portfolios dates back to the 1940s. It was not until more recently that the academic medical community embraced the use of portfolios as a learning and assessment tool in health science education. In health science education, a portfolio is a collection of documents providing evidence of learning and reflection. Portfolios are commonly used to teach and assess competencies mandated by accrediting bodies of health science programs. The goals of maintaining a portfolio may include teaching practice-based learning, professionalism, and patient care. The portfolio should establish that an individual has achieved the required standard of his or her level of training. Numerous health science undergraduate and graduate programs, including medical, nursing, dental, and pharmacy schools, utilize portfolios for these purposes. More recently, portfolios have evolved to support application for and within postgraduate educational efforts such as residency training. Finally, a portfolio can be used to facilitate job searches and interviews and for personal and professional development.[1-3] This chapter focuses on the use of portfolios to support application for a pharmacy residency.

PURPOSE OF PORTFOLIOS

Portfolios serve as a compilation of documents confirming demonstrated learning, experience, and professional growth.

Portfolios serve as a compilation of documents confirming demonstrated learning, experience, and professional growth. The portfolio can be maintained in a folder, binder, or as an electronic file. Portfolios can serve many purposes, including a record of goals and achievements, assessment of strengths and areas needing attention, collection of multiple sources of evidence documenting progress, reflection on self-growth and self-awareness, and brainstorming on ideas for future projects. In health science programs, the portfolio can be used to maintain a record of clinical experiences. Most portfolios require some indication of reflection, in which case the portfolio supports self-directed learning. A portfolio is an ever-changing document that allows an individual to be unique and highlight personal style, accomplishments, and experiences.[1-3]

The primary goal of maintaining a [professional] portfolio is to track learning and progress toward developing professional abilities or competencies.

Many colleges and schools of pharmacy across the nation utilize a *professional* portfolio to demonstrate progress in achieving ability outcomes defined for the professional curriculum. The Accreditation Council for Pharmacy Education (ACPE) provides guidelines for students to document competencies in a portfolio format during their academic education.[4] These portfolios serve several purposes. The primary goal of maintaining a portfolio is to track learning and progress toward developing professional abilities or competencies. This allows an individual to evaluate his or her accomplishments at any point in the curriculum and to identify areas needing additional attention. The second goal of the professional portfolio is to inform faculty and preceptors about a student's professional development. While the portfolio provides faculty with important feedback on curricular design and development, it also serves as a tool for the student in the residency application and interviewing process. Finally, developing a professional portfolio as a student pharmacist can ease the residency application process and/or transition to continuing professional development.[3,5,6] A *residency applicant* portfolio will likely be a modification of the *professional* portfolio that students have developed during a doctor of pharmacy program.

CONTENT: RESIDENCY APPLICANT PORTFOLIO

As previously discussed, a portfolio showcases experiences and accomplishments unique to an individual, and thus no two portfolios are alike. The content of the residency applicant's portfolio varies based on the individual and the intended use. **Table 10-1** provides an example format.

The content of the residency applicant's portfolio should begin with a table of contents and personal statement. The personal statement should include personal goals, self-assessment, and objectives for the future. This statement is a primary method by which the residency applicant shows reflection. For students applying to residency programs, a statement of short- and long-term career goals is appropriate.

The subsequent sections of a residency applicant's portfolio provide specific items that relate to the applicant's CV. The key is to provide

Table 10-1 Example Content of a Residency Applicant's Portfolio

Item	Examples
Table of Contents	
Personal statement	Personal goals, self-assessment, and objectives for the future (short- and long-term goals)
Curriculum vitae	
Certificates, honors, awards	Copies of relevant items
Representative work	Copies of projects and presentations from elective didactic courses and advanced pharmacy practice experiences that represent the quality of the applicant's work; includes elective course presentations, in-services, and presentations at local and national meetings; other items may include performance assessment forms, example monographs, completed competency checklists, SOAP notes
Scholarship	Provides any relevant research protocols, posters, publications, and newsletters
Leadership	Examples of leadership; can come from activities in organizations, committees, and community activities

documentation as well as reflection. Some sections of the portfolio should be narrative. Most narrative sections should provide reflection on a given item included in the portfolio. For example, one may provide a reflection on why the item was included in the portfolio, a summary of how the item was used (e.g., advanced pharmacy practice experience), the item's effectiveness, what has changed because of experience with the item, and what was learned by using the item, including what one learned about him- or herself. Other sections of the portfolio merely consist of the materials supplemented by a brief narrative or a rationale explaining the intent for including the document. Overall, the portfolio should provide a summary of the scope and quality of an individual's performance.

GETTING STARTED

• Characteristics of an Effective Portfolio

Portfolios will vary considerably in format; however, the most effective portfolio is well organized with a high level of documentation. The portfolio should be structured, representative, and selective. Creativity is encouraged. A portfolio should be all-inclusive—it should provide a cross section of an individual's work. Finally, the portfolio should be extremely concise with content limited only to what is required by the reviewer, while also maintaining the original intent of the portfolio.

> The portfolio should be structured, representative, and selective.

• Tips for Success

Students should start working on the portfolio early. A good filing system should be developed during an individual's training and career, and documents should be systematically collected. It is useful to review, organize, and update documents on a regular basis. Input from peers and mentors should be sought throughout the entire portfolio-building process. If the applicant's college or school of pharmacy requires a *professional* portfolio, it should be developed with residency application in mind.

• Where Things Can Go Wrong

A lack of documentation can keep vital information from being taken into consideration. The residency applicant must ensure that the portfolio matches the CV and provides examples and documentation of activities contained within that document. Excessive documentation is equally harmful. Applicants should keep in mind how the portfolio will be used. If it will be used during an interview to highlight examples of quality work, it should provide sufficient detail while avoiding superfluous material. A lack of organization and conciseness can be a critical error.

DELIVERY

Students may ask what to do with the resident applicant portfolio after it has been finalized. It is up to the applicant to decide. The portfolio's usefulness depends on its visibility. During pharmacy school, the applicant probably took the professional portfolio to the start of every new rotation. It could have served as a way to identify goals and interests, strengths and weaknesses, and, most importantly, ways to improve.[7] This process will ultimately turn residency applicants into stronger residency candidates. With modification of the professional portfolio, the residency applicant will be able to highlight why the residency program should chose him or her.

The portfolio's usefulness depends on its visibility.

As part of the search for a residency, whenever opportunities for interviewing arise, whether it is at a local or national pharmacy association meeting or an on-site interview, the portfolio should always be available. An interviewer may ask if the candidate has a portfolio, which is becoming more common. Additionally, an opportunity to show off work may arise unexpectedly. Talking about a presentation listed on the CV is not nearly as effective as pulling out a portfolio and showing it to the interviewer. Let's face it: a picture speaks a thousand words.

KEY POINTS

- A portfolio is a collection of documents providing evidence of learning and a reflective account of those documents, establishing that an individual has achieved the required standard of his or her level of training or professional development.

- The primary goal of maintaining a portfolio is to track learning and progress in developing professional abilities or competencies, allowing an individual to evaluate his or her accomplishments at any point and to identify strengths or weaknesses.

- A good filing system should be developed early in an individual's training and career, and documents should be systematically collected, reviewed, organized, and updated on a regular basis.

- The residency applicant portfolio should be structured, representative, and selective.

- The usefulness of a residency applicant portfolio depends on the user being proactive in sharing the document with others. It should be shared with preceptors and interviewers.

REFERENCES

1. Johnson PN, Smith KM. The teaching portfolio: a useful guide for pharmacists' teaching goals. *Am J Health Syst Pharm*. 2007;64:354–356.
2. Plaza CM, Draugalis JR, Slack MK, et al. Use of reflective portfolios in health sciences education. *Am J Pharm Educ*. 2007;71:article 43.

3. Buckely S, Coleman J, Davison I, et al. The educational effects of portfolios on undergraduate student learning: a best evidence medical education (BEME) systematic review. BEME guide no. 11. *Med Teach.* 2009;31:340–355.

4. Accreditation Council for Pharmaceutical Education. Accreditation standards and guidelines for the professional program in pharmacy leading to the doctor of pharmacy degree. http://www.acpe-accredit.org/pdf/FinalS2007Guidelines2.0.pdf. Accessed March 31, 2011.

5. American Society of Health-System Pharmacists. Required and elective educational outcomes, goals, objectives, and instructional objectives for postgraduate year one (PGY1) pharmacy residency programs, 2nd edition—effective July 2008. http://www.ashp.org/DocLibrary/Accreditation/PGY1-Goals-Objectives.aspx. Accessed March 31, 2011.

6. Board of Pharmacy Specialties. Portfolio requirements and scoring. http://www.bpsweb.org/specialties/scoring.cfm. Accessed March 31, 2011.

7. Accreditation Council for Pharmacy Education. Continuing professional development (CPD). http://www.acpe-accredit.org/ceproviders/CPD.asp. Accessed March 31, 2011.

CHAPTER 11

Beginning the Search for a Residency

Emily K. Flores

A journey of a thousand miles must begin with a single step.

—Lao Tzu

QUESTIONS TO PONDER

1. What should a student do at different points in the pharmacy curriculum to prepare for a residency?

2. How does a residency applicant determine the right professional position for him or her?

3. How should an applicant search for a pharmacy residency that meets his or her professional goals?

4. What characteristics should an applicant consider when considering a pharmacy residency program?

It is never too early or too late to begin considering residency training. Even if a student is not sure about a residency, it is best to research and prepare early so the student can be a competitive candidate if he or she decides to pursue a residency after graduation. Residency training may ease a pharmacist's transition from student to practitioner. The enhanced knowledge, experience, and confidence that residency training offers are some of the top reasons that students pursue residency training.[1] This chapter reviews the necessary steps to start

> It is best to research and prepare early so the student can be a competitive candidate if he or she decides to pursue a residency.

looking for a residency, which begins as early as the first year of pharmacy school. It should be considered concurrently with Chapter 15, "Choosing a Residency," when it is time to select postgraduate training.

GETTING STARTED

• Early Professional Years

When students begin their studies in pharmacy, they will inevitably begin wondering what is next; that is, what to do after graduation. A student's first step is to begin thinking about career options and interests. To learn about various options in pharmacy, students should talk with pharmacists in the community; meet with faculty mentors; enroll in postgraduate-related courses, if available; and attend sessions that their college or school may offer that describe residencies or other career paths.

Pharmacy school can be very challenging, especially adjusting to the pace and curricular content of pharmacy education during the first year. However, students must begin to build their curriculum vitae (CV) during this time (see Chapter 9, "The Curriculum Vitae and Letter of Intent," for more information). Several factors may help enhance a candidate's ability to obtain a residency.

Residency programs are looking for individuals with a professional commitment, and it is never too early to get started. There are several ways to show commitment to the profession, including getting involved in activities beyond the classroom, joining one or more professional organizations, serving on committees, and leading as an officer within the college or an organization. Pharmacy programs desire leadership qualities in residents because the goal for many residency programs is to train future leaders in pharmacy practice. Students may not know where their journey will take them yet, but it is best to be competitive for all possible options.

> Pharmacy programs desire leadership qualities in residents.

Another factor that can help a candidate stand out from others is to have research experience. Seek out an opportunity to complete a research project and present it as a poster at a local, regional, or national meeting. This research experience will be great training for the project that residents complete during residency training, and it will set applicants apart from other candidates. Students should work with faculty members at their college or school of pharmacy to learn what opportunities are available to them.

Residency applicants can strive to be competitive candidates by participating in school-level clinical competitions. Some of these competitions include the American Society of Health-Systems Pharmacists (ASHP) Clinical Skills Competition, the American Pharmacists Association (APhA) National Patient Counseling Competition, the American College of Clinical Pharmacy (ACCP) Clinical Pharmacy Challenge, and the National Community Pharmacists Association (NCPA) Pruitt-Schutte Student Business Plan Competition. These contests help refine a candidate's clinical patient care and management skills while giving them experiences to share at interviews.

Residency applicants should begin to set short- and long-term career goals early during pharmacy school to give themselves direction and to help refine their search for a position. Students should network with pharmacists and residents at meetings to learn more about pharmacy career opportunities. Students should also attend any informational sessions that their college or school of pharmacy offers on the topics of career preparation or residency training. Students should also become familiar with online resources from ASHP (http://www.ashp.org/menu/InformationFor/PharmacyStudents.aspx) and ACCP (http://www.accp.com/stunet/compass/residency.aspx) on preparation for residency training.[2]

> **Residency applicants should begin to set short- and long-term career goals early during pharmacy school.**

• Middle Professional Years

Residency applicants should continue to be involved in pharmacy organizations, service, research, and any available clinical competitions as they enter their middle professional years. If a student decides late to consider applying for a residency, he or she should strive to become involved in ways mentioned previously and take advantage of the opportunities that arise from that point forward. Residency candidates should do well in their didactic course work, ensuring that they truly learn patient care and do not study for the sole purpose of passing an examination. There is not a formal grade point average (GPA) requirement for residency training; however, it is evaluated. Students must find a good balance between extracurricular activities and their pharmacy education so they can be involved professionally but continue to do well in their studies.

> **Students must find a good balance between extracurricular activities and their pharmacy education.**

Gaining practical pharmacy work experience while in school can also set a candidate apart. Candidates must gain the number of intern hours required by the state(s) in which they plan to gain licensure after graduation. Beyond that, a candidate may be differentiated by the amount, type, or diversity of his or her internship experience. This experience will give a candidate additional patient encounters and colleague interactions to discuss at interviews.

The middle professional years are a good time for candidates to pursue research experience, if they have not already done so. This research experience sets candidates apart by giving them experience with research design, institutional review board (IRB) applications, study methods, statistical analysis, and scientific writing. Often this research can also result in a poster presentation or research presentation at a local, regional, or national meeting. This poster or presentation further sets candidates apart because they are better prepared for the research and presentation requirements of a residency.

It is during the middle professional years that students oftentimes take didactic electives and sign up for advanced pharmacy practice experiences (APPEs). Students should pick electives with their future goals in mind and choose both didactic and experiential electives that are challenging and provide diverse experiences in the practice area of interest (e.g., hospital, community, managed care, ambulatory care, etc.).

Applicants may choose to attend the ASHP Midyear Clinical Meeting (MCM) during their final didactic year to attend the Residency Showcase and get an idea of what residency training is all about. For some applicants, attending the MCM before their final year makes them more comfortable going into their final professional year. This is a great idea if the MCM is close by or if a candidate is attending for other reasons, such as to present a poster.

• Before the ASHP MCM in the Final Professional Year

Many colleges and schools provide programs that are designed to guide final professional year students through the residency selection and application process. These programs may be designed as a series of seminar sessions.[3] Alternatively, schools or colleges may decide to make information available online or through workshop settings. Candidates in their final professional year should take advantage of these information sessions or workshops to help in their preparation process.

Candidates in their final professional year should make every effort to be a part of any residency showcase events in their area. An educational institution or a local or regional chapter of a professional organization may organize and/or sponsor these events. Applicants must prepare to apply for residency positions prior to the MCM and then complete applications after the MCM in time for December to January due dates. This is the time when a candidate's research and preparation really accelerates. The first steps of preparation include having an accurate and complete CV and portfolio (see Chapter 9, "The Curriculum Vitae and Letter of Intent," and Chapter 10, "The Residency Applicant's Portfolio," for more information). Make sure to complete and submit all application materials on time and in the desired format. An increasing number of residency programs are using some form of online application, which is intended to ease application processing at the program level.[4]

> Candidates in their final professional year should make every effort to be a part of any residency showcase events in their area.

• Preparing for ASHP MCM and Other Residency Showcases

Attending residency showcases during a candidate's final professional year, whether it's a regional showcase or at the ASHP MCM, often serves as the applicant's first contact with residency programs. Candidates should take advantage of all opportunities in their local area to network with residency programs. If applicants are geographically limited, regional showcases may expose them to more programs of interest and therefore minimize the need for them to travel to the ASHP MCM.

Applicants do not need to contact programs prior to the ASHP MCM if they will be attending the meeting. If an applicant is unable to attend the ASHP MCM or chooses not to since they are applying to only a select few programs, they may wish to contact the programs around the same time of year, simply as a first contact and to let the program know to expect their application. Furthermore, candidates should not hesitate to call or e-mail a program if they have a question that cannot be answered through the ASHP or the specific program's websites.

Candidates should prepare to present themselves professionally at the ASHP MCM or regional residency showcases. Professional dress and demeanor is a necessity; this means wearing a suit, not chewing gum, and avoiding unprofessional discussions. Candidates should know which program booths they want to visit, have questions ready, take notes, and send thank-you cards to the individuals with whom they speak. Some candidates choose to have copies of their CV and/or business cards on hand to pass out at the showcase. This is optional. However, candidates should not be offended if a program requests that they send their CV with their application instead.

> **Professional dress and demeanor is a necessity.**

It is important for applicants to do their research beforehand and know whom they want to talk with while they are at the showcase. At the ASHP MCM, each program showcases only once over the course of numerous sessions, so candidates must know ahead of time which programs they want to visit at each session.

RESEARCH AND PREPARATION

Beginning with the end in mind is an important part of finding the best residency fit. When students have an idea regarding their career plans, they can begin to direct their search toward residency positions that will prepare them for their desired position.

> **Beginning with the end in mind is an important part of finding the best residency fit.**

• Type of Residency

The type of residency candidates choose to pursue is critical to preparing them for their desired career. It is important to find residency training that is both broad enough to provide all of the necessary practice experiences and tailored enough to prepare candidates for their personal career goals. Review Section I of this book for more information on various types of residencies. When candidates have an idea of potential career positions and what type or types of residencies would make them qualified for those positions, they should begin to evaluate and critique specific residency sites.

CHARACTERISTICS OF RESIDENCY SITES

All residency programs have distinguishing components, despite how similar they may seem. It is important for each candidate to find a program that is the right fit. Candidates should consider numerous issues as they narrow their residency search. If candidates are regionally limited, this will be

> **One component each candidate should consider is the strength and/or forward-thinking nature of the pharmacy leadership at the program site.**

their first degree of narrowing. If they are open to going anywhere, the following factors will help them evaluate programs and determine what is of most importance. One component each candidate should consider is the strength and/or forward-thinking nature of the pharmacy leadership at the program site.

• Size and Type of Institution

Hospital size is often described in terms of number of beds. A program may be at a 100-, 350-, or 600-bed hospital. This is a useful number when relating one residency to another because this can help candidates compare the relative size of hospitals.

A hospital may be a university teaching hospital or a community hospital. University teaching hospitals are generally larger, and pharmacy residents work alongside students and residents of other healthcare disciplines. Community hospitals may be large or small and are generally staffed by area physicians, lending themselves to a different nature of education for a pharmacy resident.

Hospitals or facilities may be evaluated by level of care in a variety of ways. A hospital may be a tertiary care center, meaning they receive cases referred from other area hospitals that do not have extensive services needed to properly care for those patients' conditions. Another distinguishing characteristic is the trauma level (highest is level 1) and neonatal intensive care unit (NICU) level (highest is NICU 3) designation of the hospital.

• Specialty Services

Hospitals may specialize in many areas of medicine. Some of the specialty services to evaluate include women's and children's services, cardiology, oncology, transplant, infectious diseases, and urgent or emergent care, among others. Candidates should make sure that their prospective programs offer the types of experiences they desire. The variety of specialty services available at a site may also relate to the availability of postgraduate year two (PGY2) residency training. If candidates are considering PGY2 training, they should determine if the PGY2 training they are interested in is available at the site they consider for their postgraduate year one (PGY1) training.

• Clinic Size and Type

When looking at an ambulatory-based residency, the clinic site is very important. Evaluate the number of providers and other residencies in other disciplines. Ascertain the role of the pharmacist as a member of the clinical care team. Candidates should think about what type of patients the clinic serves and if the patient population matches the career goals of the applicant. Many ambulatory-based residencies will offer multiple clinic sites, so make sure to evaluate all the options. If candidates are considering managed care residencies, they may consider the number of patient lives that are covered by the plan as well as the involved clinics or care sites.

• Community Pharmacy Size and Type

When looking at a community pharmacy residency, the services that the pharmacy offers will determine the resident's training. Applicants may evaluate if the site offers medication therapy management (MTM) services, immunizations, patient education programs, medication management per protocol, smoking cessation assistance, and other programs of interest. Candidates may also evaluate the number of prescriptions processed daily or weekly and whether the site is independent or part of a chain.

• Site's Professional Reputation

A site's professional reputation is one of the more difficult characteristics of a program to evaluate. Applicants may wish to speak to trusted members of their professional network and evaluate the program's current accreditation status through ASHP. New residencies are developed each year, and some of these programs may be in the early stages of the accreditation process. Some great residency programs choose not to submit for accreditation for various reasons; this makes it necessary to rely on professional networking and the track record of the program to determine if it is a good fit for the candidate.

• Number of Residents

Residency programs vary by the number of residents, ranging from 1 to more than 30. A candidate may want to be the only resident at a program so that he or she will benefit from all available resources. Others may desire a large residency class and the camaraderie that goes along with shared challenges. With larger programs, candidates may want to inquire about the program's flexibility regarding resident schedules.

• Age of Program

Candidates should consider if they prefer an established program or a program that is currently being molded. Either type of program can offer a great experience. With a more established program, residents may benefit from having preceptors that have completed a residency at that site and understand the challenges of residency. Newer programs may have the benefit of flexibility and seek resident input related to the lines of service and clinical services that are established. These young programs offer the resident a unique experience in establishing new services, which may be beneficial beyond residency.

> Newer programs may have the benefit of flexibility and seek resident input related to the lines of service and clinical services that are established.

• Required and Elective Rotations

Residency sites, especially if they are accredited, have a set of required rotations that every resident must complete. For the most part, these required rotations are similar among sites, with slight variations relative to specialty services. Candidates should be aware of these differing requirements to evaluate what training they will receive at each site.

Elective rotations allow residents to tailor their experience to their individual interests. Candidates should compare a site's available elective rotations with their desired training experiences. Electives may set a program apart from their competition.

• Preceptors

When candidates begin to narrow their residency search, they should evaluate the preceptors at the sites of interest. Many programs will provide biographical sketches of their preceptors for review, and applicants should familiarize themselves with this information before they interview at that site or meet one of the preceptors at a residency showcase. Something as simple as knowing the preceptor's specialty area can aid conversation as candidates network at showcases. A residency's preceptors determine the quality and direction of the residents' education, so a candidate's good working relationship with preceptors is important.

• Teaching and Precepting Responsibilities

Residency sites may offer a variety of teaching and precepting opportunities, and some programs offer teaching certificates. Some programs do not focus on teaching or precepting, choosing instead to focus on excellence in other areas. Some programs, however, may offer opportunities to facilitate small groups, provide didactic lectures, precept or coprecept student pharmacists, or complete a teaching certificate program. Each candidate should evaluate his or her desire to work with or teach students and what each site offers or requires in this area.

• Staffing Components

All accredited PGY1 programs have some type of staffing component, but how this is carried out can vary widely. This may be rounding on the weekend, entering orders in the central pharmacy, or reviewing clinical pharmacy consults and therapeutic drug monitoring. Evaluate the time commitment. Many programs have residents staff in some capacity every other to every third weekend, and some programs offer opportunities for moonlighting. Certain programs have residents take call on evenings, weekends, or both.[5] Another component of staffing may be responding to codes in the hospital while on duty.[6] This is a residency component that some candidates may find of great interest.

> All accredited PGY1 programs have some type of staffing component.

• Project Support and Requirements

A significant portion of residency education takes place outside of clinical patient care. These activities may include a research project, seminar, medication use evaluation (MUE), journal club, performance improvement (PI) project, administrative duties, and service to the pharmacy and therapeutics (P&T) committee. These activities are usually spread across the residency longitudinally. Sites differ in exactly what they require and how they go about assigning mentors and topics for these activities. Some sites may have a list of proposed residency projects, and others allow residents to choose their own.

NETWORKING

While candidates are evaluating all of the characteristics of various residency sites, they will begin to see the benefit of networking. Networking is an important part of a career in pharmacy and should start as early as possible. Candidates should attend meetings, make contact with professionals in their field of interest, get involved in student organizations, and hold offices or serve on committees. The earlier candidates begin building their network, the quicker it will broaden and push their career ahead. Candidates should consider some very specific networking opportunities as they journey toward their residency choice.

Networking is an important part of a career in pharmacy and should start as early as possible.

• College or School of Pharmacy Faculty

Candidates should take advantage of the professional pharmacists that are on faculty at their college or school of pharmacy. Many of these faculty members completed residency training in programs that candidates may find interesting, and mentoring by all faculty members can be a priceless part of a successful pharmacy education.

Faculty members are available from day one of pharmacy school and can provide direction to candidates along the way. Students should not hesitate to ask faculty members about their training and about residencies in general. When it comes time for references and insight into various programs, these established relationships with faculty members can be very beneficial.

• Current and Past Residents

While at the ASHP MCM and at interviews, candidates should take a special interest in learning from current and past residents. Learning about the current positions of past residents gives candidates a good idea of how a particular residency prepares residents for their desired career paths. Current residents can give candidates insight into how satisfied they have been with their residency experiences. Current residents can also share information about how much support the program offers for its residents versus how much autonomy is provided to residents. Candidates should always maintain a high level of professionalism in their conversations with current residents, while also asking all of their questions about the life of a resident at that site. Remember that current residents often have input into who is ranked in the match to replace them in the next year.

As students begin their search for a career after school, they should prepare themselves to be a competitive residency candidate. It is much better for a student to prepare early and decide later not to pursue a residency than to realize late that they did not take advantage of the time and opportunities that they had throughout school. Students should think ahead, take advantage of opportunities to learn about residency training and to network, and make sure to ask questions along the way.

KEY POINTS

- Candidates should start the process of securing a residency early to be competitive.

- Applicants should determine what type of professional pharmacist position they find interesting and then pursue residency training in that area.

- Each individual should decide what specifications are important in a residency program and use them to guide his or her search.

REFERENCES

1. Fit KE, Padiyara RS, Rabi SM, Burkiewicz JS. Factors influencing pursuit of residency training. *Am J Health Syst Pharm*. 2005;62:2226, 2235.
2. Burkiewicz JS, Sincak CA. Online tool for pharmacy students seeking residency positions. *Am J Health Syst Pharm*. 2008;65:2091–2092.
3. Bruce SP, Burkiewicz JS. Program for guiding pharmacy students through residency selection. *Am J Health Syst Pharm*. 2005;62:1488–1490.
4. Clark JS, Khalidi N, Klein KC, Streetman DD, McGregory ME, Johnston JP. Using a novel approach to collect, disseminate, and assess residency application materials. *Am J Health Syst Pharm*. 2010;67:741–745.
5. Smith KM, Hecht KA, Armitstead JA, Davis GA. Evolution and operation of a pharmacy residency on-call program. *Am J Health Syst Pharm*. 2003;60:2236–2241.
6. Toma MB, Winstead PS, Smith KM, Lewis DA, Clifford TM. Pharmacy resident participation in cardiopulmonary resuscitation events. *Am J Health Syst Pharm*. 2007;64:747–753.

CHAPTER 12

The Role of the ASHP Midyear Clinical Meeting

Larissa Hall Bossaer

You never get a second chance to make a first impression.

—**Anonymous**

QUESTIONS TO PONDER

1. What is the American Society of Health-System Pharmacists (ASHP) Midyear Clinical Meeting (MCM)?
2. Should all residency applicants go to the ASHP MCM?
3. What is the Personnel Placement Service (PPS)?
4. Should all residency applicants interview using the PPS?
5. What should residency applicants do at the Residency Showcase?

The American Society of Health-System Pharmacists (ASHP) is a national association that represents pharmacists practicing in hospitals, health maintenance organizations, long-term care facilities, home care, and other areas. ASHP hosts a number of meetings and conferences, one of which is the Midyear Clinical Meeting (MCM). The MCM occurs annually in December, and it is the largest meeting of pharmacists in the world, with more than 20,000 professionals from multiple countries in attendance. The five-day meeting serves as an opportunity for pharmacists to update their knowledge and skills on the latest in drug therapy. Other than

> The MCM occurs annually in December, and it is the largest meeting of pharmacists in the world.

educational programs, the MCM offers two major networking opportunities for residency applicants: the Residency Showcase and the Personnel Placement Service (PPS).[1,2]

The Residency Showcase is a forum that hosts hundreds of pharmacy practice residencies and over a thousand residency directors, preceptors, and current residents.[3] The showcase allows residency candidates interested in residency training to meet preceptors and residents from each residency program and learn more about the residencies and institutions themselves.

The PPS is a national recruiting event, and participation in the PPS allows prospective employees to search for positions on the CareerPharm website (www.careerpharm.com) beginning in September. Similarly, it allows potential employers to search the resumes of prospective employees. In advance of the meeting, prospective employees and employers can schedule one-on-one interviews to occur at the PPS during the MCM. Participants in the PPS range from pharmacists seeking employment in a number of settings, including hospitals and academia, to residency candidates seeking postgraduate year one (PGY1) and postgraduate year two (PGY2) residencies.[1]

> All PGY1 residencies (ASHP precandidate, candidate, or fully accredited) have the opportunity to participate in the Residency Showcase.

All PGY1 residencies (ASHP precandidate, candidate, or fully accredited) have the opportunity to participate in the Residency Showcase. Although the PPS is generally reserved for nonaccredited residencies, accredited PGY2 programs, and employment positions, there are a fair number of PGY1 programs that now use the service.

PREPARATION

In advance of the ASHP MCM, it is important to prepare. Residency candidates should plan to attend the meeting in their final professional year. Attending before the final professional year may be useful to learn more about the experience and to get comfortable with the process, but it is not required. Residency candidates should do their homework before the meeting (see Chapter 11, "Beginning the Search for a Residency," for more information). Candidates should learn as much as possible about the residency programs of interest by searching websites, requesting materials, and contacting residency directors, preceptors, and current and previous residents. They should also learn about the location, institution, rotations, requirements, specialty residency offerings, and preceptors. In advance, candidates should write down a few questions to ask the residency directors, preceptors, and current residents. Candidates should narrow the list of residency programs they want to visit to the ones for which they expect to apply. It is important to remember that there are too many residencies at the showcase to visit every booth. Therefore, candidates will want to maximize the time they spend with the residency programs that interest them the most.

It is in the candidates' best interest to join the student chapter of ASHP at their school. ASHP typically has student chapters at colleges and schools of pharmacy. Local and state chapters of ASHP can provide useful information about the MCM and connect candidates with others who are going through the same experience. By joining ASHP, candidates receive a discount on registration to the MCM, and they should register for the meeting as soon as registration opens. If candidates have advanced pharmacy practice experiences (APPEs) during the time of the meeting, they should make sure to contact their preceptor(s) well in advance and get approval to be absent for the meeting. Candidates may also have to arrange a way to make up any time that is missed.

Candidates should make hotel and travel arrangements early. The meeting typically has a host hotel that offers discounted rates, but it fills up quickly. There will be other hotels from which to choose, but candidates should not wait until the last minute to make arrangements. The longer candidates wait, the more likely their hotel will be farther away from the meeting, and it will potentially be more expensive. One way to **Candidates should make hotel and travel arrangements early.** decrease the costs of the trip is to travel with others. The meeting typically provides shuttle services back and forth among several hotels and the meeting. A shuttle route should be given to the candidate at registration, and it may be posted on the ASHP website. Map out destinations and shuttle routes before the meeting to make sure to arrive on time for events. Keep in mind that the shuttle services do not run to all hotels, so alternate transportation may have to be arranged. If candidates choose to take public transportation or taxis, bear in mind that they may run later than usual due to the volume of meeting attendees in that particular city. Therefore, candidates will need to plan ahead to arrive at the meeting on time.

Even though the Residency Showcase is considered an informal networking event, the candidate should plan to dress professionally. Men should wear suits, and women should wear pantsuits or dress suits. Plan to wear comfortable shoes to the showcase. The room is very large, and the candidate will either be walking or standing the entire time. In addition, plan to eat and drink prior to the showcase because food or drink may not be allowed in the room.

Candidates should bring their curriculum vitae (CV) and business cards, if they have them. Business cards do not need to be flashy; they need only to include the candidate's name, contact information, and identify his or her current position as either a student or resident. Exchanging business cards at the showcase has two chief purposes. It leaves a lasting impression that the candidate stopped by a particular program's booth, and it allows the candidate to get contact information of current residents or preceptors for thank-you cards. Provide a CV only if the program requests it. After exchanging business cards, candidates should take a few moments to jot down their interactions with residents or preceptors in order to personalize thank-you cards.

RESIDENCY SHOWCASE

• The Mayhem of the Residency Showcase

Before the doors of the Residency Showcase open, there will be prospective residents gathered outside anxiously waiting to enter. As the doors open, people will scurry in multiple directions. It is in the candidate's best interest to get there early. Over a thousand other residency candidates will be there seeking residencies.[3] The showcase can be overwhelming due to the sheer volume of people and information, so candidates should be prepared.

The Residency Showcase is currently held on Monday afternoon, Tuesday morning, and Tuesday afternoon, although the times and dates will likely change as the number of pharmacy residency programs continues to rise. Each residency program has only one session, so know when and where residency programs of interest will be showcasing. A residency showcase booth listing can be found online and is provided upon registration to the meeting. The listing includes all of the residencies in the showcase, along with their booth numbers and meeting times. Each booth will be different based on the program. Larger programs may be more noticeable because they generally have larger booths with many directors, preceptors, and current and prospective residents. The booths may have general informational items about the residency programs, pictures of current residents, and promotional items for the program or institution.

Come to the showcase with pen and paper, CV business cards (if used), questions about the residency program, and a positive attitude.

Candidates should come to the showcase with pen and paper, CV business cards (if used), questions about the residency program, and a positive attitude. The showcase gives the candidate a chance to learn more about a particular residency program and meet people from that program. It also gives the residency program a chance to sell the residency to many potentially exceptional candidates. Residency directors, preceptors, and current residents will try to sell the program as much as the candidates will be trying to sell themselves to the program.

• Making the Most of the Showcase

As candidates approach a booth at the Residency Showcase, they will see a table that typically has general information about the residency, along with pictures and other items. Depending on the size of the program, there will be any number of people at the booth. For larger programs, there may be the program director, several preceptors, and most of the current residents waiting to chat and answer questions. If the candidate arrives later to the showcase, he or she will likely see a massive number of prospective residents waiting in line to speak to the residency director, preceptors, or current residents, especially for the larger programs. Since there will be numerous prospective residents waiting for their chance to impress, candidates must be assertive. Candidates should be polite and professional and also watch for an opportunity to join an ongoing conversation or step forward and introduce themselves. Candidates should not be overly aggressive because this will be the first impression.

Candidates should be ready with questions (see **Table 12-1** for a list of potential questions) and get questions answered while being respectful of time. The programs see hundreds of students, so they cannot spend an hour talking to only one candidate. Practicing ahead of time may help. Ask questions that will help decide where to go for on-site interviews. The candidate should find out if the program meets their personal goals, interests, and professional values.[3]

Avoid questions that can be easily researched ahead of time, such as how many residents are in the program and the staffing requirements. During the process, candidates should find a way to make the program remember them in a good way. Have a positive, open, friendly, and professional attitude. Candidates should shake hands and introduce themselves to everyone. Maintain eye contact. Include personal interests and positive attributes in conversation with each person, and highlight any unique characteristic or distinguishing experiences. Leave a CV and business card (if used) with the program if requested, fill out an information sheet if one is available, and get a business card from each person. Make sure to thank each person for his or her time. Take a few moments after interactions to jot down a few notes. This will help to prevent all encounters from blurring together. After the showcase,

---

Table 12-1 List of Potential Questions to Ask at the Residency Showcase

To Current Residents

- What is the best aspect of your residency?
- What is the worst aspect of your residency?
- Would you do this residency over again if you had the chance?
- Do you feel that staffing opportunities help to develop your knowledge and skills as a pharmacist?
- What are your relationships with other pharmacists and healthcare professionals like?
- How are pharmacy services viewed by other healthcare professionals at your institution?
- What are your career plans after your residency?
- How do you like living in this particular area?

To Residency Directors and Preceptors

- What do you like most about working with residents?
- What are your expectations of residents at the beginning versus the end of the residency in terms of knowledge and skills?
- How do you address deficiencies in resident knowledge or skills?
- How do you provide feedback about performance to residents?

candidates should follow-up with the programs of interest by writing a thank-you card to each person who spoke with them.

PERSONNEL PLACEMENT SERVICE (PPS)

• How It Works

The PPS is not included in registration for the ASHP MCM; there is an additional registration process and fee. After PPS registration, candidates will be granted access to the online job board, where they can add their CV for prospective employers to investigate. Prospective employers or residency program directors will often contact the candidate in advance of the ASHP MCM to schedule on-site interviews. At the ASHP MCM, the candidate will have access to the PPS and will be given an electronic and physical mailbox. The mailbox serves as personal communication between the candidate and prospective employers. Prospective employers may send messages requesting interviews if this was not done in advance of the meeting. Messages may be sent to confirm interview times or as follow-up after interviews. It is in the candidates' best interest to check their mailbox multiple times during the days of PPS and respond to all messages. Even if candidates are not interested in a program or job, they should respond as a courtesy. Candidates will interview one-on-one with one or two individuals from the programs or institutions at their booth, typically behind a curtain that has a table and some chairs. The length of interviews varies by institution, but they are usually around 30 minutes.

• Pros and Cons of PPS

The PPS can be helpful in a few ways. It gives candidates more personal time with the representatives of each program or institution. Additional information may be gained by asking questions that are more revealing. It also gives candidates extra time to sell themselves as potential residents. The PPS can be particularly helpful if candidates need to narrow the focus of potential residencies or will have limited time and money for on-site interviews. It also allows candidates to interview with nonaccredited residency programs.

Unfortunately, not every residency program interviews at the PPS. The larger programs simply cannot interview hundreds of candidates during a few days. For this reason, many candidates find the PPS most useful when transitioning from a PGY1 to PGY2 residency. For many budget-conscious students, the PPS is a luxury, not a necessity, unless the candidate plans on pursing residencies that are not accredited or residencies that are exclusively in other parts of the country.

Many candidates find the PPS most useful when transitioning from a PGY1 to PGY2 residency.

Before investing time and money in the PPS, make sure that the programs of interest will be interviewing through the PPS at the MCM. Remember that it is not necessary to be involved in PPS in order to successfully obtain a residency position.

NETWORKING AND SOCIALIZING

The ASHP MCM is as much a social function as it is a business or professional function. A close and intertwined network of residency program directors and preceptors come back to the MCM year after year. This familiarity leads to friendships and networking opportunities. It is likely that a professor or preceptor that the candidate knows will have acquaintances or friends at the MCM. Additionally, it is likely that candidates will encounter recent graduates from their college or school who can introduce them to other program directors and preceptors. In other words, pharmacy is a small world. These connections may lead to invitations to formal receptions, continuing education dinners, and informal gatherings at nearby restaurants and bars. If offered, these invitations should not be declined because they can provide an insight into residency programs that cannot be gained at the showcase.

It is important to keep the small world of pharmacy in mind after the day's end. For residents, the MCM is a rare time during residency when rounds or journal clubs are not on the agenda for the following day. This allows individuals to meet up with former classmates, new colleagues, and fellow residents to have a little fun on the town. As previously mentioned, these informal encounters are excellent networking opportunities, and candidates should feel free to have fun. However, be wary of having *too much fun*. Inappropriate or unprofessional behavior can quickly undo the day's work of building a positive impression.

The ASHP MCM is a vital component in the life of both prospective residents and residency programs. Candidates should do their homework in advance and come prepared to find the right residency. Candidates should have fun but be professional and make a lasting positive impression.

KEY POINTS

- The MCM, which occurs annually in December, is the largest meeting of pharmacists in the world. It offers two major networking opportunities: the Residency Showcase and the PPS.

- The showcase allows prospective residents interested in residency training to learn more about residencies by meeting preceptors and residents, so residency candidates are highly encouraged to attend the MCM.

- Residency applicants should come to the showcase prepared to learn more about residency programs of interest, meet people from those programs, and sell themselves as exceptional candidates.

- The PPS is a national recruiting event that allows prospective residents, employees, and employers to obtain information about one another in advance and formally interview at the MCM.

- The PPS may be most useful if residency candidates want to interview with nonaccredited residencies, PGY2 residencies, or if they have limited time and money for travel to on-site interviews.

REFERENCES

1. American Society of Health-System Pharmacists. http://www.ashp.org. Accessed March 31, 2011.
2. Nick-Dart RL. How to get the most out of the ASHP meetings. *Am J Health Syst Pharm.* 2009;66:1617–1621.
3. Fotis MA. Advice for residency candidates going to the Midyear Clinical Meeting. *Am J Health Syst Pharm.* 2006:63:1787–1791.

CHAPTER 13

The Application Process

Stephen F. Eckel

Failure to prepare is preparing to fail.

—John Wooden

QUESTIONS TO PONDER

1. Has the residency applicant taken a thorough introspective review of his or her individual strengths and weaknesses?

2. Has the applicant considered all aspects of a residency program that are desirable to him or her?

3. Has the residency candidate spoken with mentors and current residents about different programs?

4. Has the applicant identified mentors who will write positive letters of recommendation?

As the prospective resident begins to prepare for the application process, it is important to recognize that this involves much more than completing the requested information and sending it to the program. If it is approached in an organized manner, the process should include internal reflection, determining the best programs to apply for, and then completing the application. The better job the candidate does of preparing to complete the application, the better the application will be. Each of these processes are further described in this chapter,

> The better job the candidate does of preparing to complete the application, the better the application will be.

with the intent of providing the applicant steps to follow to prepare the residency application.

INTERNAL REFLECTION

Having a complete understanding of oneself is essential and can provide excellent guidance throughout the process.

Finding the best residency match for a candidate can sometimes be difficult because emotions and opinions make it challenging to know where to apply. Having a complete understanding of oneself is essential and can provide excellent guidance throughout the process.[1] Candidates should think through the reasons why they went to pharmacy school and whether those desires are still relevant. If their career aims have changed, careful deliberation should ensue to understand the reasons for the different direction. Undoubtedly, most students will state they wanted to go to pharmacy school in order to serve people. However, some student pharmacists may have desires that are more specific, like assisting the underserved, owning a pharmacy, or working in a rural setting. Hopefully, the potential residents' experiential educational opportunities and elective classes have solidified their desire for residency training and affirmed their original reasons why they entered the profession.

A student pharmacist may be involved throughout pharmacy school in several activities. Items to consider include involvement with professional associations, service organizations, employment, and any other activity that is of interest. Taking time to reflect on the activities, why they were influential, and what was accomplished as a result of the potential resident's involvement is essential because this will be important when completing the residency application. This reflection should elicit thoughts and feelings about whether the activity was worthwhile, what the involvement allowed the candidate to understand about him- or herself, and whether this type of activity should be a part of the candidate's future career. Other involvement to describe, if applicable, is any leadership position held by the candidate. The inventory of activities should give the residency candidate a unique insight into his or her personality type. This will help identify what type of residency may be a better fit and the characteristics desired in a program to prepare for future career aims (see Chapter 11, "Beginning the Search for a Residency," for more information). One thing to note when developing this list of activities accomplished throughout pharmacy school is that they need to be included on the candidate's curriculum vitae (CV) (see Chapter 9, "The Curriculum Vitae and Letter of Intent," for more information).

Part of the personal inventory should include reflection on any identified or recognized strengths and weaknesses. Not only will this give candidates a better understanding of themselves and their accomplishments, but it also helps to identify any gaps or noted deficiencies in preparation for the residency interviews. For candidates who conduct this inventory before their final professional year, the list of identified gaps can be addressed before applying to residencies. For example, a student may recognize that he or she does not have any hospital work experience. This could lead the student to apply for an internship at a local hospital. A student may also recognize his or her lack of leadership experience. This could drive the student to take on larger roles in student professional associations.

The final step of the reflecting process is to share the personal inventory with mentors and close friends. Ask them for their affirmation of the list or whether their insight of the candidate's strengths and weaknesses is different. This deliberation should start a healthy and open discussion concerning others' perspective of the candidate and result in a better understanding of oneself.

The candidate should then review the various programs on the American Society of Health-System Pharmacists (ASHP) website (www.ashp.org/accreditation-residency). This site has comparative information for all ASHP-accredited programs and provides links to websites of individual programs. These websites can give much more detailed information about nuances of each residency, including career paths of past residents, descriptions of rotations and preceptors, and lists of research projects and presentations. Another potential website of interest is the American College of Clinical Pharmacy (ACCP) listing of residencies, fellowships, and graduate programs (http://www.accp.com/resandfel/index.aspx). This site includes a selective listing of both accredited and nonaccredited training programs, especially highlighting career paths for candidates who desire training in research.

After compiling the desirable activities and potential programs that have those characteristics, the residency applicant should seek advice from faculty members and past residents about their impressions of the list. Many times these individuals recommend programs based on their perception of the residency's reputation or where they completed their own training. Although this can be very beneficial, do not limit the search solely based on one individual's thoughts. There is validity to the information they share, but it is important to remember that it is their opinion.

Candidates should limit their interaction with the residency program itself to questions that cannot be answered from the information sources reviewed to date. Although contacting the program can be beneficial, it is not always helpful for candidates to e-mail residency program directors for the sole purpose of name recognition or expression of interest.

Current residents can provide updated information about the pharmacy department and the residency program that may not be listed on the website. Besides providing current insights, having the opportunity to look residents in the eye to elucidate their satisfaction can be invaluable. Current residents can give many nonverbal cues that communicate their excitement or frustration with their training experience to date. The best place for this interaction to occur is during the ASHP Midyear Clinical Meeting (MCM) or Personnel Placement Service. Although this interaction can be very helpful in affirming a candidate's decision on where to apply, it is important to recognize that everyone's training needs and strengths are different.

After proceeding through these steps, residency candidates should have six to eight programs they are extremely interested in. The completion of three or four applications was adequate in the past, but that number is increasing because most people do not get interviews at all places where they apply. The ASHP MCM will help to solidify this list by adding or removing a few programs based upon interactions there.

COMPLETING THE APPLICATION

> **Each application has different requirements, but they all have common elements.**

When the candidate has determined the programs to which he or she plans to apply, it is time to start completing the applications. Although there have been discussions of developing a common residency application for all programs, it does not yet exist. Each application has different requirements, but they all have common elements. See **Figure 13-1** for a timeline of activities.

The following items factor into each residency program application:

- *Deadline.* Application deadlines are usually in mid-December to early January during a busy time for everyone. Because of this, candidates need to budget their time well, especially since there may be delays with the

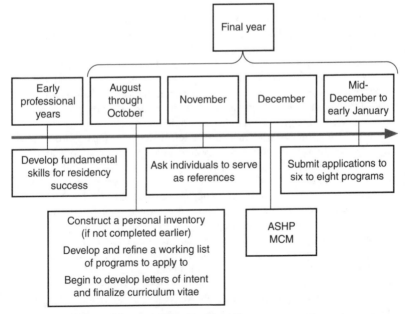

Figure 13-1: Residency Application Time Line

postal service, getting transcripts from colleges, and having mentors complete letters of recommendation. It is important to give specific instructions (e.g., required letter format, program addresses) to people who are providing recommendations and give them a deadline that will allow sufficient time for completion.

- *Directions.* Each residency program has specific directions on how to apply. For example, some programs want three letters of recommendation, and others want four. Some programs require recommendations to be completed using a standard form, and others want a traditional letter. Some programs require essays, and the prompts are never the same across programs. Other unique instructions may have an applicant collect all of the material and send it in at the same time, and other programs want to receive letters of recommendation and transcripts separately. Carefully following each program's application instructions could mean the difference between consideration and rejection.

- *References.* As mentioned earlier, applications are usually prepared and completed in mid-December to early January. Identifying references in advance is important. Potential references should be contacted before the ASHP MCM. An important consideration is who should write each letter of recommendation. Although there are differing opinions, residency applicants should strongly consider having one or two preceptors that can address clinical knowledge and skills, as well as a faculty member or a supervisor from work experience. Writing a recommendation is a learned skill, and not all pharmacists have been trained to do it well. Sometimes references never send in a recommendation letter for a candidate or, if they do, it is poorly written and does not portray the candidate in the strongest light possible. To maximize the prospective residents' chances of obtaining a well-written letter, they should choose someone who knows them well; has a positive impression of the candidate; has held faculty, leadership, or administrative positions; and is willing to spend the time needed to complete the recommendation. Failure to submit quality letters of recommendation (or any at all) is detrimental to an applicant's chance of securing a residency. After the MCM, the candidate should provide a current CV and all application instructions to the references so they will have ample time to complete the recommendation.

- *Letter of intent.* A letter of intent that is succinct, distinctive, and well written is rare among resident applicants. However, those who accomplish these goals distinguish their application from others. A standard cover letter should have a business-style header, information about the candidate, and why the candidate should be considered for the position.[2] Tailoring the cover letter to the institution is essential. Make sure to proofread the letter to remove information about other programs before sending it. See Chapter 9, "The Curriculum Vitae and Letter of Intent," for additional information.

- *Essays.* Not all applications require essays. If an essay is required, the prompts for each application will likely differ. Devoting the proper amount of effort to this part of the application may be difficult. Avoid submitting essays that have grammatical errors, are missing important concepts, or are difficult to understand. Candidates should have their mentor proofread the essay to minimize the chance for errors.

- *Curriculum vitae.* Since there is no one standard CV format, it is essential to highlight activities that the potential resident is proud to have accomplished. The CV should include advanced pharmacy practice experiences (APPEs) with good descriptors of the potential resident's experiences. It is helpful if candidates have practice sites and experiences that are similar to those of the program to which they are applying. Other important things to include on the CV are employment, organizational involvement, leadership experience, and any publications or research involvement. Distracting items to avoid are unusual fonts, floral paper, and anything else that diverts attention from the candidate's accomplishments. See Chapter 9, "The Curriculum Vitae and Letter of Intent," for additional information.

- *Transcripts.* Candidates should contact universities for their transcripts in advance so there is ample time for processing and for a program to receive the transcripts through the postal service during the holiday season.

> **Make sure there is nothing on internet social media sites, such as Facebook, that portrays the candidate in a poor light.**

Other helpful hints include following all application instructions and deadlines. Failure to do so could lead to rejection of the application. It is appropriate to contact the program to ensure that the completed application has been received. In addition, the potential resident should make sure there is nothing on internet social media sites, such as Facebook, that portrays the candidate in a poor light. Since the applicant will potentially be carrying the reputation of an institution and program into the future, compromising pictures or descriptors could deter a program from serious consideration of the candidate's application.

Finally, candidates should evaluate themselves from each residency program director's point of view to determine what each program wants in a candidate. This can be accomplished by reviewing information about the program, talking to the residency program director or current residents, or reviewing the history of the program and where previous residents are currently practicing. Potential residents should be sure their application highlights past experiences that a program director would view as an ideal fit.

Although the application process can be very stressful, it is also encouraging because it rewards candidates for all of their hard work to date. Taking the time to conduct a reflective introspection and determining what characteristics they desire in a residency program will provide candidates with essential information for completing an application. When it is completed, an application should portray the potential resident as someone who has had the experiences to be successful in the residency, and it should demonstrate that the applicant is the best choice.

KEY POINTS

- Personal reflection will help applicants understand their strengths and weaknesses; this understanding will form the basis of the residency application.

- Applicants should understand what characteristics they desire in a residency program.

- Reviewing residency websites and talking with current residents and mentors will guide candidates in developing a list of potential programs to which they should apply.

- Requesting the right people to write positive letters of recommendation is essential to a strong application.

REFERENCES

1. Teeters JL. Pharmacy residency programs: how to find the one for you. *Am J Health Syst Pharm*. 2004;61:2254–2259.
2. MIT Global Education and Career Development Center. Cover letters. web.mit .edu/career/www/guide/coverletters.pdf. Accessed March 31, 2011.

CHAPTER 14

The On-Site Interview

Anna M. Wodlinger Jackson

Make the most of yourself, for that is all there is of you.

—Ralph Waldo Emerson

QUESTIONS TO PONDER

1. Why is the on-site interview so important?

2. How should a candidate prepare ahead of time for the interview?

3. What should one expect during the interview?

4. Is there anything that should be specifically completed or avoided during the interview?

5. What is the next step after the interview is over?

After residency programs have reviewed applications, they extend offers for on-site interviews to selected candidates. Being offered an interview is an accomplishment and signifies the candidate has made it to the next round of the residency process. On-site interviews can be intimidating, and they are one of the most feared steps in obtaining a residency. This may be the first time the candidate experiences a rigorous on-site interview in a competitive environment, which can make anyone nervous. A little preparation and insight into the interviewing process can help attenuate the anxiety associated with the interview. This chapter reviews how to prepare for an interview and gives specific advice for the applicant during and after the interview.

THE IMPORTANCE OF THE ON-SITE INTERVIEW

The on-site interview is important for several reasons. It is one of the most significant factors that residency programs consider when ranking candidates.[1] It is the main opportunity that programs have to interact with candidates and evaluate their fit for the residency. The on-site interview provides an opportunity for candidates to showcase their strengths and demonstrate to the residency program why they should be chosen. For the candidate, the on-site interview provides an invaluable opportunity to evaluate the residency program in detail. It is a chance to meet with preceptors and residents to assess the residency. It also provides an opportunity to explore the location of the residency program and surrounding areas.

PREPARING FOR THE INTERVIEW

Preparation for the on-site interview is very important for success.

Preparation for the on-site interview is very important for success. There are several ways to prepare so candidates can present themselves in the best way possible. Interviewers often use the curriculum vitae (CV) to generate questions for the interview (see Chapter 9, "The Curriculum Vitae and Letter of Intent," for a detailed discussion). It is important to know every aspect of one's CV, including the particulars of all presentations, projects, and journal clubs listed. Asking questions about topics included on a CV is a way for interviewers to determine the candidate's knowledge and skills. The interviewer may also have an interest in a topic on the CV and will genuinely want to discuss it. As such, it is critical to review the CV in detail and include only the items that can be discussed with confidence. Reviewing presentation materials and journal club articles before the interview is also advisable. This is also an opportune time to review one's portfolio and included materials (see Chapter 10, "The Residency Applicant's Portfolio," for more information).

In addition to learning about the candidate's abilities and accomplishments, the interviewer wants to determine the candidate's motivation for pursuing residency training and future plans in pharmacy practice. Residency programs want residents who are enthusiastic and dedicated to the residency. Programs also want residents who have thought about their long-term career goals. This does not mean that candidates need to have exact and detailed plans for their future, but they should do some reflection and know how they will answer these commonly asked questions.

There are several other common questions that are asked during residency interviews, which are highlighted in **Table 14-1**.[1-3]

A survey of residency program interview practices found that more than 90% of 282 programs ask questions about time management.[4] Approximately 50% of programs ask questions with a clinical focus, and 9–14% of programs require a case presentation or SOAP note. The candidate should review these topics and think about how to respond to possible questions, being

Table 14-1 Commonly Asked Questions by Interviewers

- Why do you want to do a residency?

- Why do you want to do a residency with our institution?

- Where do you see yourself after a pharmacy practice residency? In five years? Ten years?

- What areas of pharmacy most interest you? Are you considering a specialty residency?

- What qualities do you possess that would make you a good resident?

- What was your favorite rotation? What was your least favorite rotation?

- Describe the most significant contribution you made to a patient's care?

- Why are you interested in our program?

- How do you handle conflict? Give me an example of a conflict you recently experienced and how you resolved it.

- What is your biggest strength? Weakness?

- Do you work better as an individual or in a group?

- Tell me about a time when you didn't have the knowledge needed to complete a task or assignment.

- Tell me about a time when you had to handle many projects or tasks at once under tight deadlines.

- Tell me in detail about a significant accomplishment in either your educational or professional career so far.

careful that responses do not sound rehearsed. Good candidates should be able to articulate why they are a strong residency candidate overall and specifically why they are a great fit for that particular program. One of the best ways to improve interviewing skills is to practice aloud with others. Some schools and professional pharmacy organizations offer mock interview sessions that allow candidates to practice interviewing. If this is not available, practicing with a friend or relative or in front of a mirror are ways to help formulate responses and improve interview skills.

Most interviewers will end a session by asking if the candidate has any remaining questions, which makes having some well-thought-out questions very important. The candidate should be prepared before the interview by researching the program, the residency site, and the preceptors. This can be accomplished by searching the residency website, doing a MEDLINE (or even Google) search on the preceptors, and asking faculty members about the program. Use this information during the on-site interview to ask specific questions that haven't been answered. **Table 14-2** provides a list of questions that candidates may wish to ask during an interview.

The candidate should be prepared before the interview by researching the program.

Table 14-2 Example Questions for Candidates to Ask During an On-Site Interview

- What are some of your former residents doing now?
- What do you consider the most important characteristic of a successful resident?
- How well are the residents' recommendations received by the staff here?
- Are there any teaching or precepting opportunities with this program?
- What presentations do your pharmacy residents conduct?
- What makes your program unique or successful?
- What do you consider the greatest strength of your program?
- What is one area of your program that you think could be improved?
- Are any major program changes planned for next year?
- How easy is it to get a specific elective rotation?
- If my practice interests change, is it possible to change my schedule or rotations?
- Are residents ever pulled from clinical rotations to cover pharmacy staff shortages?
- How are residency projects determined?

It is also acceptable to ask about something that was already discussed during the interview to clarify understanding or to express additional interest in the topic. Coming up with a question can be difficult because there is so much information already given during an interview. Therefore, preparing and knowing as much about the residency site before the interview is critical. As difficult as it may be to think of questions for each interviewer, it is important for the candidate to show the interviewer(s) that he or she is interested in the program. Candidates without questions may (rightfully or wrongfully) seem disinterested in the program compared to those who do ask.

One final thing to consider when preparing for the on-site interview is logistics. Showing up late for an interview is not the way to make a good first impression, so candidates should know exactly how to get there, where to park (if driving), and where to go for the interview inside the facility. It is a good idea to do a practice run to prevent getting lost on the day of the interview, and factor in traffic on the morning of travel. In fact, it is best to arrive early.

Showing up late for an interview is not the way to make a good first impression.

Most residency programs offer interviews beginning in mid- to late January and throughout February. If possible, candidates should try to schedule clinical advanced pharmacy practice experiences (APPEs) accordingly. Although most colleges or schools of pharmacy and APPE preceptors allow for missed days during interviews, it can become quite burdensome to miss several days of a rotation.

THE INTERVIEW

The on-site interview is typically a half-day or all-day event. Although each residency program interview will be different, there are some common elements to expect. Most interviews will start in the morning but will probably not include breakfast, so make sure to eat beforehand. All programs should include a tour of the facility that includes the various pharmacy areas as well as the clinical areas in which the residents will be practicing. Some programs may require the applicant to deliver a presentation.

The interviews themselves may vary. The different types of interviews include one-on-one interviews (one residency candidate and one interviewer) or group interviews (one residency candidate and multiple interviewers, or multiple residency candidates and one or more interviewers). Most programs will also include time spent with the current residents. Although this atmosphere may be more relaxed, it should also be considered an interview since the residents contribute input regarding applicant rankings. Some programs will require demonstration of clinical skills, including writing SOAP notes, responding to drug information questions, or doing a journal club. Although it is difficult to truly prepare for these activities before the interview, a review of some common disease states and their treatments and the proper format for a SOAP note may be helpful.

SPECIFIC ADVICE DURING THE INTERVIEW

The interview is the most significant opportunity for candidates to make an impression and convince the program that they should be selected. As such, it is important to dress and act professionally. Dress for the interview should be professional (a suit), and shoes should be somewhat comfortable because there may be considerable walking involved during the interview day. It is important to be remembered, but it is important to be remembered for something good, such as enthusiasm and clinical ability, not for being the girl who wore the leather miniskirt or the guy who talked about football the whole time. This is particularly important when spending time with the current residents because these encounters tend to be somewhat casual. Remember, any encounter with anyone in the residency program should be considered an interview and treated as such.

> Any encounter with anyone in the residency program should be considered an interview and treated as such.

Residency programs want individuals with positive attitudes. Although interviews often include questions about negative experiences, it is important to always try to stay positive in the response. Candidates are often asked to describe personal weaknesses. This should be approached as an opportunity to express how the program can help address this weakness or to turn the weakness into a strength by putting a positive spin on it. Another common question pertains to a least-favorite APPE. Candidates should respond carefully so as not to disparage the preceptor or rotation site. After all, pharmacy is a small world, and there is a high likelihood that the interviewer knows that preceptor.

During the interview, it is helpful to repeat questions back to the interviewer. This can help clarify the question and ensure that answers truly reflect what is being asked. Misunderstanding the question may result in an undesirable or unintended response. It can also allow a little more time to formulate a response. Most importantly, never guess during the interview. It is important for candidates to be honest if they cannot answer a question. If the question is about a clinical issue, it is particularly important not to guess at an answer. Interviewers understand how nervous candidates are and that candidates may not know the answer to a question. However, if a guess is made and is incorrect, it brings concern to the interviewer that the same type of response will occur with a patient when the outcome could be severely detrimental. A good response to a difficult clinical question can include a strategy for how to find the answer.

Candidates should bring a professional notebook to the interview with extra copies of their CV. The notebook can be used to record important information learned about the residency program and the names of everyone the candidate met during the interview. If a residency applicant portfolio has been developed (see Chapter 10, "The Residency Applicant's Portfolio"), it should be brought to the on-site interview, as well. Do not be afraid to ask for names or business cards for writing thank-you notes after the interview. Extra CVs give the impression of organization and can be used to help interviewers who were not given a copy before the interview.

AFTER THE INTERVIEW

Ranking residency programs can be a difficult decision, and the specific information from various residencies can become intermingled. Write down information throughout the interview to help remember key details about each program. It is important to remember the details of the residency program as well as feelings about the overall fit. Immediately following the interview, candidates should write down their thoughts about the program as a whole and with regard to meeting specific goals. When choosing a program, it is important to consider not only the opportunities provided, but also if the program's overall personality will be a good fit.

Within a week, write thank-you notes to the residency program director and interviewers. Although it is tempting and easier to send an e-mail, most interviewers appreciate the extra step that it takes to send a handwritten note. Thank-you notes should include the date the candidate was interviewed and a personalized message to the interviewer regarding a conversation or the program in general. The note should be positive and reflective of the applicant's interest in the program.

> Within a week, write thank-you notes to the residency program director and interviewers.

KEY POINTS

- The on-site interview is a great opportunity for candidates to demonstrate their strengths and interests to the residency program.

- There are several ways to prepare for an interview, and preparation is critical for success.

- It is important to stay positive during the interview and remember that all encounters with anyone from the program is part of the interview.

- It is advisable to send written thank-you notes promptly following the interview.

REFERENCES

1. Mancuso CE, Paloucek FP. Understanding and preparing for pharmacy practice interviews. *Am J Health Syst Pharm*. 2004;61:1686–1689.
2. DeCoske MA, Cavanaugh T, Elliot S, et al. A new practitioner's guide to a successful interview. *Am J Health Syst Pharm*. 2008;65:2100–2103.
3. American College of Clinical Pharmacy. Interviewing tips. www.accp.com/stunet/interviewing.aspx. Accessed March 31, 2011.
4. Mersfelder TL, Bickel RJ. Structure of postgraduate year 1 pharmacy residency interviews. *Am J Health Syst Pharm*. 2009;66:1075–1076.

CHAPTER 15

Choosing a Residency

Kelly M. Smith

Begin with the end in mind.

—**Stephen R. Covey**

QUESTIONS TO PONDER

1. What type of pharmacy career does the applicant envision?

2. Are there certain patient populations, therapeutic areas, or practice settings that are of particular interest?

3. What learning experiences suit the applicant best (e.g., longitudinal, low resident-to-preceptor ratio, certain required rotations)?

4. Which training experiences or areas of focus (e.g., teaching, formal research) does the applicant desire in a residency program?

There is no universal measure to assess a residency program's quality or its overall ranking. One way to assure that a program meets professional expectations is accreditation by the American Society of Health-System Pharmacists (ASHP).[1] Beyond that, a number of broad program features may assist candidates in selecting a residency, including the program stipend, personnel benefits, and program duration (e.g., one or two years). However, relying solely on such characteristics is shortsighted. The applicant should apply a broader lens to review potential programs in hopes of selecting the one that best fits his or her particular needs. Candidates should take

> One way to assure that a program meets professional expectations is accreditation by the American Society of Health-System Pharmacists (ASHP).

this broader evaluation approach when determining how to rank program preferences in the Residency Matching Program. The goal of this chapter is to build on Chapter 11, "Beginning the Search for a Residency," and provide guidance about how a residency applicant chooses a particular program.

NEEDS AND INTERESTS OF THE APPLICANT

The applicant must align training needs and professional interests with the features of the residency programs being considered and conduct an inventory of his or her personal and professional abilities to identify areas that require further growth and refinement. After the applicant has identified the most important elements, that list can be compared to residency programs being considered. **Table 15-1** provides a list of items an applicant may wish to consider when selecting a postgraduate year one (PGY1) residency program.

Table 15-1 Pertinent Residency Program Traits to Consider

Complete this table for each program to determine if it is a good fit.

Feature	Fit	No Fit	Notes
Skills to be acquired	☐	☐	
Pharmacy career options	☐	☐	
Area of focus (e.g., direct patient care, teaching, scholarship)	☐	☐	
Achievement of program graduates	☐	☐	
Number of residency positions (small or large)	☐	☐	
PGY2 training options in desired area of interest	☐	☐	
Nature of pharmacy practice model	☐	☐	
Integration of residents in practice model	☐	☐	
Primary patient population type(s)	☐	☐	
Type and design of learning experiences	☐	☐	
Learning experience selection, process, and scheduling	☐	☐	
Preceptors	☐	☐	
Balance of guidance and independence in resident responsibilities	☐	☐	
Preparation for teaching	☐	☐	
Engagement in teaching	☐	☐	
Drug distribution or pharmacy operations	☐	☐	
Preparation for scholarship	☐	☐	

Table 15-1 Pertinent Residency Program Traits to Consider (*Continued*)

Feature	Fit	No Fit	Notes
Engagement in scholarship	☐	☐	
Program accreditation status	☐	☐	
Program setting (e.g., academic medical center, community pharmacy, clinic, industry)	☐	☐	
Geographic location	☐	☐	
Stipend, benefits, and cost of living	☐	☐	
Other feature:	☐	☐	
Other feature:	☐	☐	
Other feature:	☐	☐	
Other feature:	☐	☐	
Other feature:	☐	☐	

ASSESSING INDIVIDUAL NEEDS

The list of program features that should be evaluated during the pharmacy residency selection process is long. However, the applicant should not overlook certain key elements.

• Motivations for Seeking Residency Training

The applicant should determine the types of skills he or she desires to acquire during residency training. If becoming a clinical faculty member is the target career goal, training in and experience with clinical teaching, as well as classroom instruction, would be features to seek in a residency program. The applicant should also consider the type of pharmacy position he or she wishes to secure after completion of the program. For instance, developing services and measuring their impact on care are important skills to develop if the applicant wishes to secure a clinical coordinator position.

• Program Setting

Some applicants have geographical constraints that will limit their ability to relocate beyond a certain area. A candidate without such limitations should carefully consider his or her willingness to move to a specific location. Beyond geography, consider a desire to practice in a particular patient care setting, whether that is a community hospital, academic medical center, physician's office, community pharmacy, industry, or other facility.

• Individual Program Considerations

Many applicants find they perform better if they can train alongside a large number of other residents; thus, programs that offer multiple positions may be more desirable. Others may feel more comfortable in a small program. If a postgraduate year two (PGY2) residency is desired, a practical consideration for many applicants is the likelihood that they could remain at the training site to complete a PGY2 program. Perhaps even more important than areas of practice focus is the institution's mission in residency training. If a site is committed to preparing residents to enter practice with a generalist skill set, this program may not be well suited for a candidate who foresees a career as a faculty member or clinical specialist. Candidates should investigate a program's track record to learn the career paths of its previous residents.

The commitment of the pharmacy department or group to the residency program can be a very important consideration. The greater the program is integrated into the unit's function, the greater the focus on the program and the commitment to its success.

• Program Focus

Residency programs are composed of a number of required learning experiences (e.g., specific rotations, projects). In addition to determining if the program offers the types of rotations or learning experiences that meet specific interests or needs (e.g., adult critical care, pediatrics, geriatrics), the applicant should assess the capacity of the program to meet his or her unique interests and its ability to accommodate interests that may change throughout the residency year. One practical consideration is the ability of the site to schedule rotations in the resident's area(s) of interest early in the residency year. Such an approach may assist in confirming or ruling out an applicant's interest in pursuing a PGY2 residency or employment position in that area of focus before the onset of the recruitment season.

• Preceptors

Working alongside a number of individual pharmacists exposes the resident to different training and practice styles, which should contribute to creating an approach that suits the resident's personal needs. Thus, a program with numerous preceptors is often attractive to candidates. Beyond the numbers, consider the style of guidance. If an applicant's experience with rounding to provide direct patient care is minimal, pursuing a program that expects residents to practice independently early in the residency may be a poor match.

• Additional Learning Experiences

A strong foundation in pharmacy operations (i.e., drug distribution process) is critical to a successful pharmacy practice, regardless of the specific setting or individual's job responsibilities. Thus, the applicant should work to gain experience in this area, even if he or she does not foresee a career that directly involves dispensing medications. Most residency programs involve the resident in the operations of the unit. Evaluate this involvement to determine if programs provide a sufficient grounding in and experience with operations. Is the pharmacy sufficiently equipped with contemporary technology, from automated medication preparation and dispensing equipment to electronic medical records? A lack thereof may not prepare the resident well for a future position in a setting with an extensive technology infrastructure.

Many residency candidates have some interest in teaching or guiding student pharmacists as an element of their own careers (see Chapter 21, "Teaching Responsibilities"). The applicant should explore such an interest thoroughly and determine if the residency programs being considered offer extensive opportunities to precept students in the practice setting. Many residencies also afford additional opportunities to teach students, including those in other healthcare professions, in the classroom setting. Preparation for such teaching may be integrated throughout the residency or be delivered in a teaching skills development program (i.e., teaching certificate program). Such formal training in teaching techniques is valuable even outside of a formal academic position because sound instructional principles can be applied to a number of common pharmacy encounters (e.g., patient counseling, in-service education). In addition to teaching, the applicant may wish to gain more experience in the area of scholarship (see Chapter 22, "Scholarship Responsibilities"). Examining the extent to which a program's preceptors are involved in scholarship is generally a good indicator of the site's emphasis on the development of a resident's scholarly abilities.

THE END IN MIND

Completing a residency is an investment in one's professional future. Selecting a residency with the right fit may be just as critical, if not more so, as the application or interview processes. Although ASHP-accredited residencies boast common outcomes for their trainees and work from a well-defined set of goals for residents, they may vary significantly in their structure, design, and features. Thus, it is important to determine the elements that are most important to select the program with the best fit. Most important is identifying programs that will best prepare the candidate for future professional achievements, which can be achieved by approaching the selection with the end in mind.

> It is important to determine the elements that are most important to select the program with the best fit.

KEY POINTS

• Congruency between the residency candidate's needs and interests and the residency program's features should be the primary consideration in selecting a residency program.

• To determine critical elements in the residency evaluation process, first conduct an inventory of personal and professional abilities and identify areas that require additional experience and training.

- Delineate professional desires, optimal learning styles, and potential future areas of specialization to determine which programs meet specific interests.

REFERENCE

1. American Society of Health-System Pharmacists. ASHP regulations on accreditation of pharmacy residencies. http://www.ashp.org/s_ashp/docs/files/RTP_ResidencyAccredRegulation.pdf. Accessed March 31, 2011.

CHAPTER 16

The Residency Matching Program

Michael A. Crouch

I find that the harder I work, the more luck I seem to have.

—Thomas Jefferson

QUESTIONS TO PONDER

1. Who administers the pharmacy Residency Matching Program?
2. Is the match required for all ASHP-accredited residencies?
3. How difficult is it to obtain a residency through the pharmacy match?
4. Are there ways to secure a residency without going through the match?
5. What is the *scramble*?

The American Society of Heath-System Pharmacists (ASHP) is the accrediting body for pharmacy residencies. It has used a matching system for about two decades, most recently administered by the National Matching Service (NMS).[1,2] The purpose of the match is to coordinate the selection process between applicants and residency programs. The rationale behind the development of the match is that it levels the playing field and allows applicants and programs to rank their preferences concurrently after sufficient time for on-site interviews.[2] In March 2007, ASHP expanded the matching program to include all ASHP-accredited residency programs rather than just first-year offerings.[3]

The pharmacy match applies to accredited postgraduate year one (PGY1) and postgraduate year two (PGY2) residencies. Exceptions may include U.S. Department of Defense and U.S. Public Health Service Commissioned Corps positions.[4] The match includes residency programs that are precandidate, candidate, or fully accredited. A new program may choose to delay the submission for precandidate status and thus select its resident(s) outside of the matching process the first year the residency is offered. In such situations, the applicant is strongly encouraged to determine the residency program's ultimate goal regarding accreditation, which can be retroactive for current resident(s). To determine the accreditation status of individual programs, consult the ASHP Residency Directory, available online at http://www.ashp. org/ResidencyDirectory.

Although ASHP sponsors and supervises the match, NMS administers it annually. The pharmacy match is similar to other matching programs administered or sponsored by the NMS, including residencies in dentistry, psychology, neuropsychology, osteopathic medicine, and medicine. Of the matching programs administered by the NMS, the pharmacy match is the second largest.

OVERVIEW OF THE MATCH

The process of the residency match starts with applicants and residency programs applying to participate. Residency programs apply to take part in the match in August the year before the residency start, whereas resident candidates apply by the following January. It is critical for applicants to know that the deadline to submit for the match is mid-January of the year they plan to secure a residency.

Applicants must consider various issues when trying to secure a pharmacy residency and are encouraged to study all chapters in Section II of this book, paying particular attention to Chapter 12, "The Role of the ASHP Midyear Clinical Meeting"; Chapter 13, "The Application Process"; and Chapter 14, "The On-Site Interview." The pharmacy match coordinates only the placement of the applicant—it does not manage applications or on-site interviews. Applicants determine which programs they wish to consider, submit application materials directly to individual programs (typically due from mid-December to early January), and set up interviews if they are offered by the institution. Interviews occur in January, February, and potentially early March.

Applicants and residency programs submit their rank order lists to NMS in early March. The applicant's rank order list specifies the programs he or she would like to attend, if selected. The residency program provides a comparable list of applicants they will accept. The rank order lists from applicants and residency programs provide preferences, rated from the most to least preferred. When completing the rank order list, applicants should list their true preferences and avoid ranking programs by how they think programs will rank them. Importantly, applicants should list only the programs they are committed to attending since the match results are a binding agreement. The program must offer the position to the match applicant and the applicant must accept. Only through written agreement by both parties can an applicant or program withdraw after the match, which is infrequent.[4]

After submission of rank order lists, NMS uses the stated preferences to place individuals into a residency position. Algorithms place applicants based on mutual preferences, and an applicant cannot match with a program that he or she did not list. During the matching process, an applicant might not match with a particular program on his or her list for two main reasons: the program did not rank the applicant, or positions were filled with higher-ranked applicants. The NMS website provides further details regarding the computer process, examples, and common misunderstandings (http://www.natmatch.com/ashprmp).[4]

> Importantly, applicants should list only the programs they are committed to attending since the match results are a binding agreement.

IMPORTANT DATES

Applicants and residency programs must apply to participate in the match, and there are a number of key dates to keep in mind. Individual residencies complete program agreements in August of the year prior to the start of the residency program, and NMS provides a list of available programs in November. Although applicants can register for the match as early as August of the year prior to starting a residency (most residencies start in July), the applicant must sign up by mid-January (consult the NMS website for the exact date, since it varies from year to year). The time required for applicants to receive their match number may be delayed, so applicants are encouraged to enter the match as soon as they plan to pursue a residency to ensure that the match number is available when applications are due. See **Table 16-1** for a list of key match dates.[4]

Table 16-1 Key Dates Related to the Match

Date	Activity
August	NMS match registration opens.
November	Match website provides a list of participating programs.
January	Recommended date by which applicants register for the match (consult the NMS website for the exact date).
Early March	Final date for submission of applicants and program rank order lists (consult the NMS website for the exact date).
Late March	Results of the match are released. A listing of unfilled positions is provided for the scramble.
Late March to late April	Program directors send letters of confirmation to match applicants for their signature.
July	Start date for most residency programs.

Source: Adapted from American Society of Health-System Pharmacists. ASHP residency matching program. http://www.natmatch.com/ashprmp/index.htm. Accessed March 31, 2011.

EARLY COMMITMENT

For individuals currently enrolled in a PGY1 residency, an early commitment process provides a mechanism by which they can secure a PGY2 position within the same organization. For this to occur, six criteria must be met[4]:

1. The program has a formal, written policy to promote PGY1 residents.

2. The PGY2 program is registered in the match.

3. The applicant is enrolled in a PGY1 residency offered by the same sponsor of the PGY2 program.

4. Residency program directors (RPDs) for both the PGY1 and PGY2 residency sign a letter of agreement that commits the PGY2 position to the applicant.

5. The PGY2 program pays the nonrefundable fee to the NMS.

6. The agreement letter is signed by both parties, and the NMS fee is paid by mid-December (the exact date varies by year).

There are pros and cons related to early commitment. The major advantage to the resident is that he or she secures the position before the ASHP Midyear Clinical Meeting. This can relieve significant stress to all parties involved. Conversely, early commitment may hinder the resident candidate from pursing all PGY2 options. Given the timing of the early commitment process, the resident may have completed only three rotations in his or her PGY1 residency before formally applying to stay a second year, and the resident may not have had adequate time to determine if that site is where he or she would like to complete a second year.

Programs cannot attempt to use the early commitment process to secure an applicant for a PGY1 program. Conversely, a new residency program that has not submitted for precandidate status will not participate in the pharmacy match and can make offers at any time. If this is the case, the applicant is strongly encouraged to determine the residency program's ultimate goal regarding accreditation.

THE SCRAMBLE

Applicants should realize there are unfilled positions every year after the match, and they should continue to seek a residency through the scramble.

After release of the match results in late March, there will be unfilled residency positions. The *scramble* is the time when unmatched residents apply for unfilled positions.[5] The NMS immediately provides the list of unfilled positions to applicants and programs who did not match. Applicants should realize there are unfilled positions every year after the match, and they should continue to seek a residency through the scramble if they were unable to secure a position through the match. The scramble entails programs and applicants directly contacting one another. Importantly, the match ends in late March, and

NMS and ASHP have no role in the scramble. This is a very hectic time, and those seeking a residency through the scramble should be proactive and contact programs with unfilled positions promptly. A mentor or advisor at the college or school can be a tremendous asset during this time. Depending on the program, there may be a modified application process that entails a phone interview, on-site interview, or both. For those who enter this phase, interviews and offers can occur at any time, and programs often fill open positions within days.

PREVIOUS MATCH RESULTS

The number of applicants seeking a pharmacy residency continues to increase annually. Conversely, there are not a sufficient number of PGY1 residency slots currently available to meet the demand. Previous match results are available on the NMS website (http://www.natmatch.com/ashprmp). The match results vary from year to year, but two important themes have developed. First, the number of positions filled through the match consistently occurs at a high rate (> 90%), whereas the number of applicants securing a program through the match is decreasing (< 65%).

KEY POINTS

• The NMS administers the match under the sponsorship and supervision of ASHP.

• To secure an ASHP-accredited residency program, applicants must participate in the match.

• Accredited PGY1 and PGY2 residencies must go through the match process.

• Applicants currently enrolled in a sponsor's PGY1 residency may secure a PGY2 residency at the same organization through the early commitment process.

• Applicants who do not secure a residency through the match are encouraged to participate in the scramble and apply for unfilled positions.

REFERENCES

1. King DL. Planning for the ASHP resident matching program. *Am J Health Syst Pharm*. 1995;52:1863–1864.
2. Lifshin LS, Teeters JL, Bush CG. ASHP resident matching program: how does it work? *Am J Health Syst Pharm*. 2004;61:446.
3. Teeters JL. New ASHP pharmacy residency accreditation standards. *Am J Health Syst Pharm*. 2006;63:1012–1018.
4. American Society of Health-System Pharmacists. ASHP resident matching program. http://www.natmatch.com/ashprmp/index.htm. Accessed March 31, 2011.
5. Crannage AJ, Drew AM, Pritchard LM, Murphy JA. Managing the residency scramble. *Am J Health Syst Pharm*. 2011;68:110, 114.

Making the Most of a Residency

Mollie A. Scott, Section Editor

■ Checklist: Excelling in a Pharmacy Residency

Overall, a successful resident shows the following characteristics:

- Accepts criticism
- Adaptable
- Assertive
- Attentive
- Collegial
- Committed
- Cooperative
- Curious
- Decisive
- Dedicated
- Dependable
- Efficient
- Embraces change
- Energetic
- Enthusiastic
- Ethical
- Humble
- Independent

- Informed
- Motivated
- Optimistic
- Organized
- Patient centered
- Positive
- Proactive
- Professional
- Punctual
- Reliable
- Resourceful
- Respectful
- Sincere
- Strong work ethic
- Tactful
- Team player
- Trustworthy
- Understanding

Complete this checklist to ensure excellence during a residency. (Note: The acronyms are defined at the end of the checklist.)

Before the Residency

❑ Obtain your pharmacy license promptly.
❑ Complete any unique program requirements (e.g., credentialing for Veterans Administration).
❑ Write a mission statement (personal values, professional passions).
❑ Assess your individual strengths and areas to improve (reevaluate your time-management skills).
❑ Review the residency manual in-depth, if available.
❑ Sign up for residency rotations, projects, and/or longitudinal experiences, if possible.

July–September

❑ Sign up for residency rotations, projects, and/or longitudinal experiences, if they are still pending.
❑ Establish specific residency goals and evaluation points in conjunction with the RPD.
❑ Review evaluation forms used by the residency program.
❑ Finalize dates, mentors, and deadlines for major activities, where applicable:
  - Residency project (identify advisor)
  - Continuing education program (identify advisor)
  - Manuscript (if required)
  - Case conference and/or journal club
  - Didactic teaching
  - Experiential teaching
  - Medication use evaluation
  - On-call program
  - Staffing
❑ Enroll in a teaching certificate program, if available and relevant to your career goals.
❑ Begin project development and submit it for IRB approval (likely requires training course).

October–December

❑ Complete your quarterly residency evaluation (revise your goals as necessary).
❑ Receive IRB approval and implement your residency project, including data collection.
❑ Begin the process of determining the next step after your residency (e.g., PGY2 or position).

- ❑ Attend the ACCP Annual Meeting (in October), if it is relevant to your program or career goals.
- ❑ Attend the NCPA Annual Meeting (in October), if it is relevant to your program or career goals.
- ❑ Attend the ASHP Midyear Clinical Meeting (in December), if it is relevant to your program or career goals.

January–March

- ❑ Complete your quarterly residency evaluation (revise your goals as necessary).
- ❑ Finalize your residency project and prepare for presentation at the regional residency conference.
- ❑ Begin manuscript preparation, if required.
- ❑ Participate fully in the recruitment of the resident(s) for the next year.
- ❑ Submit applications for the next step after your residency (e.g., PGY2 or position).
- ❑ Attend the APhA Annual Meeting (in March), if it is relevant to your program or career goals.

April–June

- ❑ Complete your quarterly residency evaluation (revise your goals as necessary).
- ❑ Attend, network, and present your residency project at the regional residency conference.
- ❑ Attend the AMCP Annual Meeting (in April), if it is relevant to your program or career goals.
- ❑ Attend the ACCP Spring Meeting (in April), especially if you are seeking board certification.
- ❑ Disseminate your residency project findings (e.g., poster, publication, etc.).
- ❑ Complete your final residency evaluation.

Acronyms

ACCP: American College of Clinical Pharmacy
AMCP: Academy of Managed Care Pharmacy
APhA: American Pharmacists Association
ASHP: American Society of Health-System Pharmacists
IRB: Institutional review board
NCPA: National Community Pharmacists Association
PGY2:   Postgraduate year two
RPD: Residency program director

■ Key Readings Related to Excelling in a Pharmacy Residency

Clinical Pharmacy in the United States

Elenbaas RM, Worthen DB. *Clinical Pharmacy in the United States.* Lenexa, KS: American College of Clinical Pharmacy; 2009.

Leadership and Self-Deception: Getting Out of the Box

The Arbinger Institute. *Leadership and Self-Deception: Getting Out of the Box.* 2nd ed. San Francisco, CA: Berrett-Koehler Publishers; 2010.

StrengthsFinder 2.0

Rath T. *StrengthsFinder 2.0.* New York, NY: Gallup Press; 2007.

The 7 Habits of Highly Effective People

Covey S. *The 7 Habits of Highly Effective People.* Rev ed. New York, NY: Free Press; 2004.

The 21 Irrefutable Laws of Leadership

Maxwell JC. *The 21 Irrefutable Laws of Leadership: Follow Them and People Will Follow You.* 10th rev anniv ed. Nashville, TN: Thomas Nelson; 2007.

The Five Dysfunctions of a Team

Lencioni P. *The Five Dysfunctions of a Team.* San Francisco, CA: Jossey-Bass; 2002.

Who Moved My Cheese?

Johnson S. *Who Moved My Cheese?* New York, NY: G P Putnam's Sons; 1998.

CHAPTER 17

What to Expect Throughout the Year

Michael A. Crouch

Success usually comes to those who are too busy to be looking for it.

—Henry David Thoreau

QUESTIONS TO PONDER

1. How should a resident plan for a successful year?

2. What is the usual time commitment associated with a residency program?

3. What are the typical residency requirements?

4. When do specific residency activities normally occur throughout the year?

5. How do expectations differ between postgraduate year one (PGY1) and postgraduate year two (PGY2) residencies?

After an applicant has secured a residency, apprehension and uncertainty may build as the start date approaches. Most residency programs require residents to be licensed promptly, and the process to attain or transfer a license should begin immediately when an individual has secured a residency. Some programs may also require credentialing (e.g., Veterans Administration), and the soon-to-be resident should address this immediately, if applicable. A successful transition from student to resident entails multiple issues; hard work and thinking and acting like a pharmacist are key aspects. Most residents appreciate the greater autonomy that comes with

A successful transition from student to resident entails multiple issues; hard work and thinking and acting like a pharmacist are key aspects.

the position, but such opportunity also carries greater responsibility. The residency program director (RPD) will likely afford independence to residents from day one, but usually the level of autonomy grows throughout the year as the resident gains credibility with the RPD and preceptors.

Residency training is a bridge from being a student to becoming a clinical professional. An approach that helps residents make this transition has been coined LOGIC (learning, organization, goals, independence, and communication).[1] This concept entails maintaining the high level of knowledge gained in pharmacy school, learning time management and prioritization skills, setting short- and long-term goals, developing self-reliance, and tailoring verbal and written communication skills. Good planning is essential because "a successful residency year does not just happen; you have to work at it."[1]

The resident should plan to spend long hours at the site to take advantage of this accelerated learning environment.

Many residency program directors equate a single year of residency training to at least three years of working as a pharmacist. As such, the residency year can be stressful because it requires a heavy workload and a steep learning curve. The resident should plan to spend long hours at the site to take advantage of this accelerated learning environment. The work schedule and hours will vary from one residency to the next, but the American Society of Health-System Pharmacists (ASHP) has adopted the Accreditation Council for Graduate Medical Education (ACGME) policy regarding duty hours. According to these standards, resident duty hours are limited to 80 hours per week (including on-call activities) *averaged* over a four-week period.[2] Updated ACGME requirements were released in 2010 for implementation in 2011. These recommendations further clarify requirements in the areas of supervision, workload, maximum hours per week, maximum length of duty period, in-hospital on-call frequency, minimum time off between scheduled duty periods, maximum frequency of in-hospital duty, mandatory off-duty time, moonlighting, duty hour exceptions, and home call.[3]

OVERVIEW OF THE YEAR

Orientation with the RPD should happen early in the program, allowing for clarification of expectations and review of unique requirements of the individual residency program.

Residents will likely receive a residency manual when they arrive to start the program, or they might receive it beforehand as part of a welcome packet. The manual provides an overview of the program, and residents need to take time to familiarize themselves with the document. Particular areas that require focused attention include general residency requirements, resident expectations, and human resource issues. Residents should also consider the structure of the residency program, including to whom they directly report. Orientation with the RPD should happen early in the program, allowing for clarification of expectations and review of unique requirements of the individual residency program.

The residency year begins with an orientation, likely one to three weeks in length. Depending on the number of residents in the program, it may be an individual or group orientation. The orientation acquaints the resident with the institution and outlines the expectations beyond the residency handbook. **Table 17-1** provides typical requirements of a residency program. Expectations will vary greatly based on the healthcare environment, including the hospital, community pharmacy, long-term care facility, ambulatory care clinic, and managed care organization, among others.

During orientation or soon thereafter, the residency program may select a chief resident. A recent survey demonstrates that 28% of residency programs have a chief resident, resident-in-charge, or comparable leadership position; oftentimes, larger programs (e.g., four residents or more) create this position.[4] The duties of a chief resident include serving as a liaison between the residents and the resident program leadership and coordinating meetings, educational programs, and schedules. For residents that are interested in this opportunity, it provides a mechanism by which to develop and enhance leadership skills.[4]

After orientation, the residency year is oftentimes divided into quarters, with a major separation point between the first and second half of the year being the December ASHP Midyear Clinical Meeting. See the checklist titled Excelling in a Pharmacy Residency on page 135 to identify when certain program requirements likely occur. Certain required activities will

Table 17-1 Typical Requirements of a Residency Program

Case conference and/or journal club

Clinic involvement and required longitudinal experiences

Clinical rotations (required and elective)

Continuing education program

Didactic teaching

Experiential teaching

In-services

Involvement in a peer-review process (e.g., journal article review)

Major residency project

Management and leadership development

Manuscript for publication

Medication use evaluation

On-call activities

Staffing

Teaching certificate*

*Many residency programs offer a teaching certificate. Although it is often optional for PGY1 residents, it may be required for PGY2 residents. At this time, there is no accrediting body for teaching certificates.

happen throughout the year, such as rotations, on-call responsibilities, longitudinal experiences, and staffing. Conversely, the timing of other activities requires scheduling, such as didactic and experiential teaching, continuing education programs, and case conferences and journal clubs. When signing up for these activities, residents are encouraged to consider dispersing the requirements throughout the year.

The first half of the residency program (July to December) entails learning the pharmacy system and organization and developing plans for the year (see Chapter 19, "The Residency Evaluation Process," to understand how evaluations will occur throughout the program). Residents are strongly encouraged to be proactive during this stage and seek feedback from preceptors and the RPD.

Planning is critical to being successful in a residency program.

Planning is critical to being successful in a residency program. Depending on the program structure, residents may be assigned to different mentors (e.g., research advisor, continuing education mentor, etc.) who help facilitate major program requirements and provide guidance for planning the residents' next career steps. Necessary planning may include the development and implementation of a lecture, research project, continuing education program, medication use evaluation, and manuscript for publication. The resident handbook will provide the exact requirements of the program, and good preparation is necessary to ensure completion of all program requirements.

The second half of the residency year (January to June) often entails implementation and finalization of major requirements. The second half of the year fully implements the residency project, medication use evaluation, and manuscript. This is a very busy time for residents, and success during this part of the program directly relates to earlier planning.

From December to March of the residency year, residents play a pivotal role in residency recruitment for the following year. Recruitment includes attendance and participation at the ASHP Midyear Clinical Meeting in December, which may include organizing the Residency Showcase and Personnel Placement Service (PPS). In January and February, residents will likely help select candidates for interviews and facilitate on-site visits. In early March, the residency selection committee will determine which individuals to list on the rank order list for the National Matching Services, usually with input of the current residents.

In addition to the previously discussed resident-specific requirements, the resident will be involved in other activities during the year. Some residency programs have a residency trip, which may include a visit to ASHP headquarters (Bethesda, Maryland), other residency programs, or both. These trips are oftentimes a unique blend of business and fun and serve to build camaraderie within the residency class in addition to being a good learning opportunity.

Residents will also attend a regional resident conference in the second half of the year. Seven residency conferences occur annually, including

Eastern States, Great Lakes, Midwest, Midsouth, Southeast, Southwest Leadership, and Western States.[5] The physical location of the residency program determines which conference residents attend. The primary purpose of residency conferences is to present research projects (poster or platform presentation) and to network with other residents and residency programs.

Residency programs seeking ASHP accreditation follow numerous steps to apply for, attain, and maintain accreditation. Residents may be involved in one or more of these steps, depending on the status of the program. Residents entering a newly established residency program will likely be very involved in the application process. For established programs, accreditation occurs at least every six years. Potential resident involvement in this process includes completion of presurvey questionnaires (due 45 days before the survey visit), the residency survey visit (usually two days), and response to the formal team report from ASHP.[6] The ASHP Commission on Credentialing reviews the site specific survey and recommends the accreditation status and length of accreditation. This long process requires the participation of residents and is a great way for residents to learn more about residency training and accreditation.

IMPORTANT DIFFERENCES BETWEEN RESIDENCIES

What to expect throughout the year depends on the type of residency program. Program expectations for hospital, community pharmacy, ambulatory care, and managed care residencies have inherent differences. These differences were likely part of the candidate's rationale to apply for specific residency programs. Irrespective of the chosen path for additional training, the rationale to complete any type of postgraduate residency revolves around a sincere desire to excel as a clinician and to provide high-quality, direct patient care.

There are notable differences between postgraduate year one (PGY1) and postgraduate year two (PGY2) residency programs. Advanced PGY2 residences are the penultimate training ground to develop a clinical pharmacist. As such, the level of autonomy is markedly higher in PGY2 residencies as compared to PGY1 residencies. Moreover, the PGY2 program traditionally focuses on a specialized area of practice, such as critical care or cardiology. Staffing requirements may differ in PGY2 residencies, which include no staffing to alternative staffing models that include weekdays and/or weekends. Given the focus of the residency program, staffing may occur in a specialized area or satellite pharmacy. Another notable difference between programs is the presentation of the residency project. Although PGY2 residents may attend regional conferences, their research may also be presented at a specialty conference.

The level of autonomy is markedly higher in PGY2 residencies as compared to PGY1 residencies.

Many individuals completing a pharmacy residency program, particularly PGY2 residencies, will choose a career path that includes teaching responsibilities in the didactic or experiential settings, or both. Therefore, completion of a teaching certificate is an important component of a residency program to prepare residents to assume this educator role, and it may be a requirement of PGY2 programs.

KEY POINTS

- Good planning is the key aspect for success in a residency.

- Residents should embrace the long work hours as a necessary part of training.

- Program expectations will vary greatly based on the residency program healthcare environment (e.g., hospital, community pharmacy, ambulatory care clinic, managed care organization).

- PGY2 residents have increased autonomy and likely have increased teaching requirements.

REFERENCES

1. Lieberman-Blum SS, Kang L, Kugler A, Khalifa M, Schiller DS. Making the most of your residency. *Am J Health Syst Pharm*. 2008;65:293–295.
2. Smith KM, Trapskin PJ, Armistead JA. Adoption of duty-hour standards in a pharmacy residency program. *Am J Health Syst Pharm*. 2005;62:800–803.
3. Nasca TJ, Day SH, Amis ES. The new recommendations on duty hours from the ACGME task force. *N Engl J Med*. 2010;363(2):e3.
4. Burkiewicz JS, Bruce S. Chief resident in pharmacy residency programs. *Am J Health Syst Pharm*. 2007;754–761.
5. American Society of Health-System Pharmacists. Regional resident conferences. http://www.ashp.org/menu/Residents/GeneralInfo.aspx. Accessed March 31, 2011.
6. DeCoske MA, Bush PW, Teeters JL. Preparing for pharmacy residency accreditation surveys. *Am J Health Syst Pharm*. 2010;67:469–475.

CHAPTER 18

Developing a Personal Mission and Leadership Style

Mollie A. Scott

It's not about how to achieve your dreams. It's about how to lead your life. If you lead your life the right way . . . the dreams will come to you.

—**from** *The Last Lecture* **by Randy Pausch**

QUESTIONS TO PONDER

1. How can a resident use a personal mission statement to achieve professional goals?

2. Why is it important for residents to identify their professional strengths and weaknesses?

3. What are strategies that residents can use to assess and improve their leadership skills?

When a new resident has begun training, it is time to begin asking what's next. It may feel overwhelming to start thinking about the next career steps when the dream of becoming a resident has just been realized. Residents may have spent a great deal of time meticulously plotting the steps that it took to complete the pharmacy degree, while others perhaps simply fell into pharmacy as a career choice without a great deal of planning. Regardless of the intensity of previous planning, it is important for residents to identify long-range career goals beyond the residency. By focusing on the future early in the

> By focusing on the future early in the residency year, the resident can make wiser choices about mentors, electives, and residency projects.

residency year, the resident can make wiser choices about mentors, electives, and residency projects. In addition, it is important for residents to begin to evaluate their individual strengths and weaknesses, since a good understanding of oneself is the foundation for effective leadership. This chapter reviews tips for developing a personal mission statement and identifying preferences for leadership styles, both of which are important building blocks for successful self-leadership.

DEVELOPING A PERSONAL MISSION STATEMENT

In his book *The 7 Habits of Highly Effective People*, author Stephen Covey outlines the importance of beginning with the end in mind (**Table 18-1**).[1] Beginning with the end in mind, or Habit 2 of the 7 Habits, Covey teaches us to set our sights on what it is that we ultimately want to accomplish.

Covey challenges us to identify the most important roles that we play in our lives and in the lives of others and encourages us to develop a personal mission statement so that our dreams are achieved for each of these roles. To do this, the resident should spend a quiet afternoon alone reflecting about what is important in his or her life. Begin writing the personal mission statement by asking the following questions:

- What are my gifts?

- What are the guiding principles in my life?

- Who are the most important people in my life?

- What makes me go home at the end of the day and say, "That was a great day!"

- What is my dream position after residency?

- What do I want people to say about me at my retirement party?

There are no dos or don'ts for writing a personal mission statement; residents should use their own personal style as they organize it. After answering

Table 18-1 *The 7 Habits of Highly Effective People* by Stephen Covey
Habit 1: Be proactive
Habit 2: Begin with the end in mind
Habit 3: Put first things first
Habit 4: Think win–win
Habit 5: Seek first to understand, then to be understood
Habit 6: Synergize
Habit 7: Sharpen the saw
Source: Adapted from Covey SR. *The 7 Habits of Highly Effective People*. New York, NY: Free Press; 2004.

the questions in the previous list (and any others that come to mind), it is time to draft a statement that summarizes a personal mission. Options for expressing a personal mission are limitless; missions may be stated in one sentence or a lengthy narrative. Residents that are more artistic may choose to draw or paint a picture that characterizes their mission.

When composing the personal mission statement, do not focus just on what is important professionally; after all, there are many aspects to people outside of being a pharmacist. Each of us is endowed with special gifts, and it is up to each of us to identify our gifts, develop them fully, and use them to have a positive impact on the lives of our patients. Developing a mission statement that integrates both personal and professional lives can help residents understand the importance of seeking a work–life balance. Residents may wish to seek out mentors who effectively model balancing professional activities with their personal lives. Maintaining personal interests and hobbies during residency is important. For instance, residents who love to sing might seek opportunities to join a local choir, whereas a newly married resident might develop goals that are focused on nurturing the new marriage. Incorporating personal responsibilities and interests into the mission statement is a good way to ensure that professional goals are not achieved at the expense of personal relationships.

A personal mission statement based on personal values, professional passions, and strengths can serve as a compass during everyday work life as well as during future career decisions. The personal mission statement should complement the goals that the resident and the residency program director (RPD) set at the beginning of the residency year. Residents should consult their personal mission statement before applying for a new position and identify those organizations most in line with their values and goals. When interviewing for a position, ensure that the responsibilities of the position and the culture of the organization are in sync with the personal mission statement. If the position matches well with the mission statement, this may be the perfect place to begin a career in pharmacy. If not, it may be better to keep looking. As residents graduate and move on with their careers, they may find it helpful to review their personal mission statement at the start of each year to ensure that they are still headed toward their big-picture professional goals and are maintaining a work–life balance. Practicing pharmacy without a personal mission statement is like driving in an unfamiliar city without a GPS: a destination will eventually be reached, but it may not be the intended place.

> A personal mission statement based on personal values, professional passions, and strengths can serve as a compass.

DEVELOPING A LEADERSHIP STYLE

Much of the residency year focuses on developing critical thinking skills and applying knowledge to the care of individual patients to ensure positive drug therapy outcomes. Residency

> The first step in developing strong leadership skills is to assess and appreciate personal strengths and weaknesses.

training should also include opportunities for self-reflection, development of self-awareness, and self-management skills. Covey teaches that no one is effectively able to manage time, but we can all learn to effectively manage ourselves.[1] The first step in developing strong leadership skills is to assess and appreciate personal strengths and weaknesses. Two tools that have been used successfully in leadership development are the 360° feedback process[2] and the Myers-Briggs Type Indicator (MBTI).[3]

An effective way to identify personal strengths and weaknesses is to participate in a 360° feedback process.[2] Key elements of the 360° feedback process are described in **Figure 18-1**.

During the 360° feedback process, team members (including preceptors, resident colleagues, and others) complete an anonymous survey that objectively assesses leadership talents and areas for growth while also providing concrete behavioral examples. This exercise is completed separately from the formal residency evaluation processes. An important component of the 360° feedback process is the resident's honest self-evaluation. Remember, the purpose of this exercise is to increase leadership effectiveness, not to tear down

Figure 18-1: Key Elements of the 360° Feedback Process

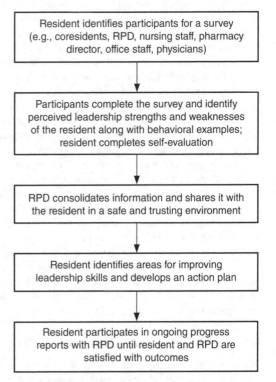

Resident identifies participants for a survey (e.g., coresidents, RPD, nursing staff, pharmacy director, office staff, physicians)

↓

Participants complete the survey and identify perceived leadership strengths and weaknesses of the resident along with behavioral examples; resident completes self-evaluation

↓

RPD consolidates information and shares it with the resident in a safe and trusting environment

↓

Resident identifies areas for improving leadership skills and develops an action plan

↓

Resident participates in ongoing progress reports with RPD until resident and RPD are satisfied with outcomes a resident's confidence. The RPD compiles the information from all those who were surveyed and then reviews the results with the resident in a safe, trusting environment. Areas of weakness that are identified by others but not previously identified by the resident may be a blind spot and can hopefully lead to a moment of epiphany on the part of the resident. The positive feedback provided by team members can reaffirm those strengths that the resident has identified and can be encouraging when the going gets tough.

The resident selects several specific areas to focus on for a period of time (e.g., a month, a quarter) and develops specific measurable objectives and a learning activity to assist with improving a given area. For instance, if the resident identifies that conflict resolution is challenging, he or she might choose to read a leadership book about dealing with conflict and discuss it with the RPD. If the resident learns that the tone of his or her e-mails have created barriers to communication with others, the resident may focus on the wording of e-mails or talking by phone to avoid misperceptions. The most important thing is to approach this process with an open mind and to embrace the leadership truth that we cannot effectively lead others if we are unable to lead ourselves. To lead ourselves, we must first understand our strengths and weaknesses and seek to build on our strengths and improve in areas that do not come as naturally.

> We cannot effectively lead others if we are unable to lead ourselves.

Another effective leadership development tool is the MBTI (**Table 18-2**).[3] The MBTI is a tool that can identify natural preferences for leadership styles. Isabel Briggs Myers, a developer of the MBTI, stated, "Whatever the circumstances of your life, the understanding of type can help make your perceptions clearer, your judgments sounder, and your life closer to your heart's desire."[3]

The MBTI identifies four specific areas of preferred characteristics:

1. *Extroversion or Introversion (E or I)*: Describes preference to focus on the outer or inner world

2. *Sensing or Intuition (S or N)*: Describes preference for taking in information

3. *Feeling or Thinking (F or T)*: Describes how decisions are made

4. *Judging or Perceiving (J or P)*: Describes preferences for planning

Having the residency team (RPD, preceptors, and residents) complete an MBTI training workshop together with a trained facilitator can help each team member identify their preferred working styles. Moreover, understanding the type of each team member can lead to a deeper appreciation of what others have to contribute and potentially avoid conflict in the workplace by promoting better understanding of each other's strengths. Each team member learns what type they naturally prefer (one of 16 types identified by four letters, such as ENFJ, ISTP, etc.). Residents learn more about how they make decisions, how they are energized, and their preferences for planning, which can increase leadership effectiveness.

Table 18-2 Myers-Briggs Type Indicator Preferences

E–I dichotomy

Extraversion (E) — People who prefer extraversion focus on the outer world of people and activity; they gain energy from interacting with others.

Introversion (I) — People who prefer introversion focus on their own inner world of ideas and experiences; they receive energy from reflection.

S–N dichotomy

Sensing (S) — People who prefer sensing take in information that is real and tangible; they are attuned to practical realities.

Intuition (N) — People who prefer intuition take in information by seeing the big picture; they are attuned to seeing new possibilities.

T–F dichotomy

Thinking (T) — People who prefer thinking in decision making look at the logical consequences of choices and actions; they are energized by analyzing problems.

Feeling (F) — People who prefer feeling in decision making consider what is important to them and others involved; they are energized by appreciating and supporting others.

J–P dichotomy

Judging (J) — People who prefer to use their judging process like to live in a planned, orderly way, seeking to regulate and manage their lives; they like to make decisions and move on.

Perceiving (P) — People who prefer to use their perceiving process like to live in a flexible, spontaneous way, seeking to experience and understand life instead of control it; detailed plans feel confining.

Source: Adapted from The Myers & Briggs Foundation. The MBTI instrument for life. http://www.myersbriggs.org/. Accessed March 31, 2011.

KEY POINTS

- Begin the residency year with the end in mind.

- Develop a personal mission statement based on professional interests, personal strengths, and personal values.

- Seek ways to develop leadership skills, such as completing a 360° feedback process and the MBTI.

REFERENCES

1. Covey SR. *The 7 Habits of Highly Effective People.* New York, NY: Free Press; 2004.
2. Edwards MR, Ewen AJ. *360° Feedback: The Powerful New Model for Employee Assessment and Performance Improvement.* New York, NY: AMACOM; 1996.
3. The Myers & Briggs Foundation. The MBTI instrument for life. http://www.myersbriggs.org/. Accessed March 31, 2011.

CHAPTER 19

The Residency Evaluation Process

Freddy M. Creekmore

If you don't know where you are going, you will probably end up somewhere else.

—Laurence J. Peter

QUESTIONS TO PONDER

1. How does one establish personal goals for a residency program?
2. What are the expectations of a residency program director (RPD)?
3. How can goals be accomplished during the year?
4. Can goals change throughout the residency program?
5. How will an RPD ensure that expectations are met during the year?

Evaluation is vitally important in a residency program because it ensures the quality of educational components. Evaluations can be difficult for the evaluator and the person being evaluated, but if they are organized properly from the outset, they can be done efficiently and effectively. When preceptors systematically document a resident's achievement of goals, the evaluation process can be a rewarding experience. The purpose of this chapter is to build on the residency outcomes listed in Section I and show how goals are used to meet these educational outcomes.

DETERMINING PURPOSE AND SETTING GOALS

The most important part of the evaluation process is to determine what will be evaluated. The resident should be evaluated on how well he or she achieves the goals of the residency program. Careful selection and understanding of the goals at the outset is critical. The goals should be part of an individualized residency plan specific to each resident.

Before setting goals, the resident, program director, and potentially other major preceptors should discuss the overall purpose of the residency, which will help establish goals. So that each understands the other better, determining the purpose of the residency from the resident's perspective and from the RPD's perspective is important before the process of evaluation begins.

Residencies accredited by the American Society of Health-System Pharmacists (ASHP) have well-defined evaluation terms. In that context, the term "outcome" is the broadest. For postgraduate year one (PGY1) residencies there are six required outcomes.[1] Under each outcome there are 1 to 12 goals. ASHP utilizes the Residency Learning System (RLS), which organizes each goal into several educational objectives.[2] ASHP also provides instructional objectives under each educational objective as examples of how a resident might demonstrate competence for the corresponding objective. It should be noted that activities are different from goals or objectives. Activities are learning opportunities and occasions for the resident to demonstrate accomplishment of a goal. See **Table 19-1** for an example of how all these items relate to one another.

For residencies not accredited by ASHP, the terms may be used differently or not at all. It is vitally important that the resident and the RPD understand the purpose and goals of the residency, as well as how the resident will show that he or she has accomplished these goals.

At the beginning of the residency, after discussing the purpose, the resident and the RPD must determine all the outcomes, goals, and objectives that will be addressed during the residency. This will be the master list. For ASHP-accredited PGY1 residencies, the first six outcomes along with all their associated goals and objectives are required (see Section I of this book, "The Case for Pharmacy Residencies," for details regarding outcomes of individual residency programs). There are elective outcomes beyond those required for specific programs. It is important that the resident and the RPD review those outcomes and determine which to include in the evaluation process. Elective outcomes can be added later during the residency if the RPD and the resident believe it is appropriate. For instance, one of the elective outcomes for ASHP-accredited PGY1 hospital-based residencies is to participate in the management of medical emergencies. At the beginning of the year, it may be decided that the resident will not be required to do this activity and will therefore not be evaluated on it. Perhaps after six months

Table 19-1 An Example of an ASHP Outcome, Goal, Objectives, and Associated Activity

Outcome	Provide evidence-based, patient-centered medication therapy management with interdisciplinary teams.
Goal	Collect and analyze patient information.
Educational objective	Collect and organize all patient-specific information needed by the pharmacist to prevent, detect, and resolve medication-related problems and to make appropriate evidence-based, patient-centered medication therapy recommendations as part of the interdisciplinary team.
Instructional objective	Identify the types of patient-specific information the pharmacist requires to prevent, detect, and resolve medication-related problems and to make appropriate evidence-based, patient-centered medication therapy recommendations as part of the interdisciplinary team.
Activity	During the acute care internal medicine rotation, monitor patients prior to interdisciplinary rounds daily and use the information gathered to improve patient care while on rounds. Formally present examples to the preceptor on a weekly basis.

Source: Modified from American Society of Health-Systems Pharmacists. Resident's guide to the RLS, third edition. http://www.ashp.org/DocLibrary/Accreditation/ResidentsGuidetotheRLS.aspx. Accessed March 31, 2011. Reprinted with permission.

the resident completes a critical care rotation and decides that he or she would like to participate on the hospital's cardiac arrest response team. At that time, it would be appropriate to add the proper outcomes.

In addition to the elective outcomes listed by ASHP, the RPD and the resident may have additional goals they wish to add. These should be discussed and clearly described at the beginning of the program. Ultimately, the RPD and the resident should arrive at a residency plan that includes customized goals for each resident.

Understanding the purpose of the residency and setting appropriate goals is vital to the evaluation process. If the goals are overly ambitious, residents will feel as if they are failing and will become discouraged. If the goals lack rigor, then residents will not be driven to attain their potential and may become complacent. While it may be difficult to determine the perfect set of goals at first, with reassessment and adjustments on a regular basis, the right balance can be reached.

> Understanding the purpose of the residency and setting appropriate goals is vital to the evaluation process.

DETERMINING WHERE AND WHEN GOALS WILL BE ADDRESSED AND ASSESSED

After the goals have been established and mutually agreed upon, the resident and the RPD should decide what components of the residency address each goal and would therefore best assess the resident's progress toward those goals. Assigned preceptors should evaluate residents via learning experiences, each having at least one goal assigned to it, and each goal should be assigned to at least one experience during the residency year. Most parts of the residency will have multiple goals, and most goals will be assigned to multiple learning experiences throughout the year. For example, under the outcome "manage and improve the medication-use process," one of ASHP's required goals is to "prepare and dispense medications following existing standards of practice and the organization's policies and procedures." This goal would be assigned to the distributive staffing component of the residency. It may also be assigned to a learning experience where dispensing medications is part of the daily practice.

From the master list of goals, it is imperative to create a subset of goals for each separate learning experience of the residency. Each activity is an opportunity to develop, so the resident must understand the key skills being taught or refined. The RPD should take goals directly from the predetermined master list of goals established previously (see the ASHP website for a detailed listing of goals: http://www.ashp.org/s_ashp/docs/files/RTP_PGY1GoalsObjectives.doc). For each individual rotation and other learning experiences, the resident should be evaluated on his or her progress toward the goals assigned to that component.

THE ASSESSMENT OF PROGRESS TOWARD MEETING GOALS

Each learning experience of the residency should have a designated preceptor to oversee that part of the residency and to evaluate the resident's progress toward the assigned goals. Designating a preceptor for formal presentations, for research projects, and for staffing is highly recommended for a complete, comprehensive, and organized evaluation. The RPD may need to serve as the preceptor of some of these items, but having a separate presentation mentor, research advisor, and staffing supervisor is a great way for a resident to learn from different pharmacists with different styles.

The resident should meet with each preceptor at the start of each learning experience and review the goals for that component of the residency. The preceptor should explain the activities in which the resident will participate in order to achieve the goals for that part of the residency. Furthermore, the preceptor should describe what criteria will be used to assess the resident's progress toward the goals and to determine whether the resident has met the goals.

As an example, one of the goals for an inpatient medical service rotation is "design evidence-based monitoring plans." The learning experience preceptor should explain to the resident how he or she will be monitoring patients on a daily basis and perhaps the requirement that twice weekly the resident will need to describe in writing a current patient case, including a problem list, monitoring parameters, assessments, and a therapeutic plan for each problem. The preceptor should give the resident feedback on each written case. At the end of the rotation, the preceptor will determine whether the resident has met the goal or has made satisfactory progress toward the goal based on the documentation of cases the resident provided throughout the rotation.

In the previous example, the preceptor gave the resident formative and summative evaluations. Formative evaluations are those meant to improve a resident's performance on that particular component of the residency. Not all formative evaluations need to be written. Informal, oral formative evaluations should be given frequently. Formal written formative evaluations should also be utilized. Residencies accredited by ASHP may use a type of formative assessment called a *snapshot*, which is a written formative evaluation of a particular outcome or goal.[2] These are documented discussions with the resident regarding the resident's progress toward each of the goals. The discussions can be held as frequently as is appropriate and are especially helpful when a resident is struggling to meet a particular goal.

> Formative evaluations are those meant to improve a resident's performance on that particular component of the residency.

Summative assessments for rotations or other components of a residency are judgments of how well the resident progressed toward the goals during that experience or in the program. For ASHP-accredited residencies, the terms *Needs Improvement*, *Satisfactory Progress*, and *Achieved* are the preferred choices. Unlike formative assessments, they should always be written and sent to the RPD. Even though they are summative, the resident should still try to learn from the evaluation and improve when the next opportunity arises.

> Summative assessments for rotations or other components of a residency are judgments of how well the resident progressed toward the goals during that experience or in the program.

It is crucial that the RPD meet and evaluate the resident every two to three months, often referred to as the quarterly evaluation. Before that meeting, the resident should assess his or her progress toward all program goals. It is important to take the self-assessment seriously. Residents should record ways they are doing well in a particular area and areas for improvement. Self-assessment will help residents visualize what they have accomplished and understand what they still need to do.

Before the quarterly evaluation, the RPD should read and analyze each evaluation completed by all residency preceptors and the self-assessment done by the resident. Often it will include evaluations from the resident's longitudinal clinic preceptor, research preceptor, presentations preceptor, academic teaching preceptor, staffing preceptor, and potentially others. The RPD may serve as one or more of these preceptors and should perform evaluations in those roles in addition to the RPD evaluation. Each quarter,

Each quarter, the RPD should evaluate the resident's progress toward the master list of goals for the residency. the RPD should evaluate the resident's progress toward the master list of goals for the residency, taking into account all the evaluations from all the different preceptors. Until the final evaluation at the end of the residency, all the quarterly evaluations are formative, but they are formative for the residency as a whole. The last evaluation by the RPD is summative, and at that time the resident must have met all the required goals of the program. The purpose of the summative evaluation is to evaluate all of the program goals and decide whether the resident is able to complete the program. The other meetings, including the first meeting, should be long working meetings where a great deal of detailed evaluation, reflection, and planning takes place.

At each of the formal quarterly formative evaluation meetings, the resident and the RPD should accomplish several things. The RPD should discuss the evaluations from other preceptors with the resident and give the resident an opportunity to respond. Goals that the resident has already achieved and no longer need to be evaluated should be identified. Goals for which the resident is not making satisfactory progress need to be discussed in detail, and a plan should be formulated for how the resident will improve. The resident and the RPD should make sure all the goals are still relevant and remove any goals that are not. Likewise, new goals should be added that may have arisen since previous quarterly meetings. In addition, project deadlines for the next quarter should be set.

REACTION TO ASSESSMENTS

Residents need to learn how to react to positive and negative evaluations. Occasionally a preceptor will simply heap praise on a resident because they do not want to offend the resident. Although praise is helpful and appropriate, each evaluation should identify something a resident can do better. If the preceptor does not offer that, the resident should request it.

Residents must not take criticism personally. Residents must not take criticism personally. When a critical comment is offered from a preceptor on a particular goal, it is sometimes easier to go quickly to the next goal; however, residents should strive to thoroughly understand why their performance is lacking and what they can do to improve. Just telling a resident to improve in an area or try harder is insufficient. Preceptors should offer specific advice on what to do differently. Again, if the preceptor does not offer this criticism and advice, the resident should request it.

Although it is infrequent, there may be an occasional unfair evaluation by a preceptor. The resident should discuss the evaluation with the preceptor in a calm and professional fashion. If the resident still believes the evaluation was overly harsh, he or she should write an explanation of why the evaluation is overly critical and forward that explanation to the RPD. The RPD should meet with the preceptor and decide how to proceed. The evaluation might not change, but the RPD should give the resident an opportunity to meet the goals associated with that component of the residency with a different preceptor. Each situation is different and each must be dealt with on an individual basis.

Sometimes a preceptor may deliver an evaluation that is so brief in its comments that it does not aid the resident's development. Even worse is when a preceptor fails to formally evaluate the resident at all. In both cases, the resident is justified in asking the preceptor for some, or for additional, formal feedback. Normally a preceptor will take time to give formal feedback to the resident when it is respectfully requested. It is unacceptable for a preceptor to remain part of a residency program if he or she will not provide adequate evaluations.

RESIDENT'S EVALUATIONS OF THE RESIDENCY PROGRAM

A resident should be given the opportunity to evaluate individual preceptors, rotations, the site or sites, the RPD, and other components of the program, as well as the program as a whole. Residents should take these evaluations seriously. Preceptors and the RPD will discuss these evaluations, and improvements can be made based upon them.

Oftentimes, the evaluation can improve the program for the current resident. For instance, if the resident states in an evaluation that a preceptor did not explain the goals of the rotation at the beginning, the RPD may speak to that preceptor and describe the importance of appropriately orienting the resident to the rotation.

Sometimes an evaluation from a resident may affect future residents in that program. For example, a resident may state in an evaluation of the residency site that the office space for the residents was inadequate. The RPD may show that evaluation to department administrators and acquire additional or improved office space for future residents.

DOCUMENTING ACHIEVEMENT OF GOALS

Documenting progress toward, and achievement of, the goals of the residency is crucial. ASHP-accredited residencies use forms provided in their RLS system or use an online evaluation tool. The online tool ResiTrak is available to ASHP-accredited residencies free of charge from ASHP.[3] The software program automates all evaluation processes described in this chapter. If the online tool is not used, residencies should develop forms and tools to effectively document formative and summative assessments of each component of the residency and the resident's overall progress toward the identified goals.

> Documenting progress toward, and achievement of, the goals of the residency is crucial.

In addition to forms, residents should accumulate documentation of accomplishments, projects, and other residency-related items. All of this documentation should be collected in the resident's notebook. Traditionally, this documentation is kept in a loose-leaf binder with an assortment of dividers and pages, but the entire notebook could be kept electronically. The resident's notebook should contain the following:

- All evaluations completed during the residency
- Copies of presentations and lectures
- Feedback from students under the resident's supervision
- Copies of written manuscripts of grant proposals and committee presentations
- Examples of patient care plans
- Other documents deemed necessary by the resident and the RPD to thoroughly capture the resident's achievement of all the program goals

Although they are often feared, evaluations of residents are critical and need not be considered onerous. A well-designed system of evaluation based on predetermined, and often reassessed, goals should guide the resident toward achievement of those goals. Program directors, preceptors, and residents should utilize the evaluation system to improve performance and refine the skills of all involved.

KEY POINTS

- Residents should determine their personal goals for the residency program.
- Establishing a clear understanding of the expectations of the RPD at the beginning of the program is crucial to every resident's success.
- Seeking and receiving frequent and detailed feedback regarding progress toward goals is essential to achieving program outcomes.
- It may be necessary to adjust goals throughout the year.
- The RPD will obtain feedback about a resident's progress from many sources, including the resident; residents should listen attentively to all of the evaluations and work with the RPD to ensure achievement of all expectations.

REFERENCES

1. American Society of Health-System Pharmacists. Required and elective educational outcomes, goals, objectives, and instructional objectives for postgraduate year one (PGY1) pharmacy residency programs, 2nd edition—effective July 2008. http://www.ashp.org/s_ashp/docs/files/RTP_PGY1GoalsObjectives.doc. Accessed March 31, 2011.
2. American Society of Health-System Pharmacists. Resident's guide to the RLS, third edition. http://www.ashp.org/DocLibrary/Accreditation/ResidentsGuidetotheRLS.aspx. Accessed March 31, 2011.
3. American Society of Health-System Pharmacists. ResiTrak. http://www.ashp.org/s_ashp/docs/files/rtp_resitrakhandout041907.pdf. Accessed March 31, 2011.

CHAPTER 20

Clinical Service Responsibilities

David W. Stewart

No enterprise can exist for itself alone. It ministers to some great need, it performs some great service, not for itself, but for others; or failing therein it ceases to be profitable and ceases to exist.

—Calvin Coolidge

QUESTIONS TO PONDER

1. How did pharmacy transition from a product-based to patient-centered profession?

2. What are the usual clinical service responsibilities of a pharmacy resident?

3. What do patients expect from healthcare professionals?

4. What attributes make a resident responsible and professional?

5. In the future, how will pharmacists provide care?

In the nineteenth century, a drugstore was similar to the description that many of today's patients might give a local pharmacy. Although medications were dispensed, the main business was in merchandising. The turn of the twentieth century brought about the legal requirement that pharmacists receive formal education and be licensed, and hence the profession began to evolve. During the 1960s, pharmacists transitioned from merchandisers to clinicians, and pharmacists in various settings began providing an increased level of patient care.[1] This movement started what we now call *clinical pharmacy*, a term poorly defined and often misunderstood outside of the profession.

Today there is the expectation that pharmacists provide more than a product, and current advances within the profession have established avenues of reimbursement independent of the products provided. Students recite an oath as they enter into the profession, pledging to achieve outcomes, care for patients, and "embrace and advocate changes that improve patient care."[2] As pharmacists embark on their career, they should keep in mind that others have pioneered and laid the groundwork for clinical pharmacy as we know it today. Following in their footsteps, pharmacists should remember the traits of professionalism. The following list is 10 traits of a professional, which was used to spearhead the American Pharmacists Association's development of professionalism among pharmacists and students[3]:

- Knowledge and skills of a profession
- Commitment to self-improvement of skills and knowledge
- Service orientation
- Pride in the profession
- Covenantal relationship with the patient
- Creativity and innovation
- Conscience and trustworthiness
- Accountability for his or her work
- Ethically sound decision making
- Leadership

New residents should consider how to incorporate these ideas into clinical service, service to organizations, service to the profession, and community service. This chapter focuses on the most important service provided by pharmacists: direct patient care. Residents should also endeavor to become active members of the profession during their residency training on local, state, and national levels.

PROVISION OF PATIENT CARE

The profession of pharmacy and healthcare has evolved over the past five decades.

Pharmacists are now recognized in many settings as an integral part of the healthcare team. New pharmacy residents should note that in the history of medicine and pharmacy, pharmacists have not always been active participants at the patient's bedside. The profession of pharmacy and healthcare has evolved over the past five decades, and evidence supports the utility of pharmacist-provided, patient-centered care. Many new residents

Table 20-1 Example Clinical Service-Related Activities

Medical attending rounds

Clinical case discussions

Cardiac arrest rapid response team

Consults

Drug therapy reviews

Grand rounds

In-services

Immunizations

Medication reconciliation

Medication therapy management

Patient counseling

Pharmacotherapy clinic

Pharmacokinetic monitoring

will now easily integrate into established pharmacy service lines and interact naturally with other patient care providers, such as physicians, nurses, and allied health professionals. **Table 20-1** provides examples of clinical services residents may undertake, depending on the type of practice site. It should be noted that postgraduate year two (PGY2) residents have greater autonomy to address clinical activities with more limited preceptor oversight. Some residents, however, may face the same barriers that their preceptors dealt with to establish themselves as part of these activities, so it may be necessary for residents to discuss with their preceptors how they can effectively integrate into the healthcare team.

PHARMACIST–PATIENT INTERACTIONS

There are numerous ways residents or practitioners should conduct themselves in the presence of patients. Depending on cultural and generational differences, certain things that residents would not consider to be offensive could offend the patient. The key point is to follow the golden rule: do unto others as you would have them do unto you. Manners should not be checked at the door when entering the practice site, and pharmacists should always put their best foot forward with patients (as well as with other professionals). Always ask permission before addressing or examining a patient. Introduce yourself by both name and title while clearly displaying an identification badge. Address patients by their surname unless a patient grants permission to do otherwise.[4] When patients are sick they seek out healthcare professionals, and pharmacists must act professionally to be identified in a professional way.

When patients are sick they seek out healthcare professionals, and pharmacists must act professionally.

PHARMACIST–HEALTHCARE PROFESSIONAL INTERACTIONS

In situations where there is a structured medical team (e.g., institutional pharmacy or ambulatory care), the medical team is much like a military unit where individuals have defined roles. There is a definite hierarchy of discipline and order. Ultimately, the attending physician is responsible for all decisions and is legally liable. The medical residents are his or her assistants, and some carry more responsibility than others. Senior medical residents may be responsible for other medical residents, overseeing them in the day-to-day operations. The medical students are normally ardent learners gleaning as much knowledge as possible. They may have some basic responsibilities for a limited number of patients. Other healthcare professionals are critical members of this team and include allied health professionals and midlevel practitioners, such as nurse practitioners and physician assistants, case managers, and respiratory therapists.

One might ask how pharmacists fit into this equation. Pharmacists typically serve as consultants and may exercise this function in numerous modalities. In some settings, pharmacists may provide direct patient care. The role varies from one setting to the next, but pharmacists must fit within established schemes. Representatives of the pharmacy profession may include the pharmacist (sometimes referred to as the *pharmacy attending*), a pharmacy resident, and pharmacy students. In this model, the pharmacy resident will be depended on; however, respect from other professionals, including pharmacist preceptors, physicians, medical residents, and even students, must be earned over time.

> **If pharmacists want to be treated as legitimate members of the team of healthcare professionals, they must act as professionals.**

Despite the hierarchy with one individual being ultimately responsible (the attending physician), this scheme should also be visualized as a team effort. When disagreeing with a decision, one should address the issue with the utmost humility and respect, always addressing more senior individuals in a formal manner. Likewise, pharmacy residents should respectfully address pharmacist preceptors formally, especially in front of the medical team. If pharmacists want to be treated as legitimate members of the team of healthcare professionals, they must act as professionals and promote the profession while completing their duties.

Although pharmacy residents may serve as consultants, this does not imply that they should provide quality pharmaceutical care only when specifically consulted. A good pharmacist provides comprehensive support to each member of the team and will likely have valuable insight and knowledge to contribute to the care of each patient. Communicating recommendations appropriately is a major determinant in whether or not care plans are implemented. In fact, the best care plans could fail to be implemented because inappropriate communication is used during the process, and this is detrimental to both the patient and the profession.

One crucial factor for success in communicating care plans is to communicate with the correct person at the correct time. For example, it is usually best to first communicate with the medical resident who is directly responsible for the care of the patient. Only if the patient is still not receiving appropriate care would one escalate up the chain of medical command to the senior medical resident(s) and then lastly to the attending physician. Surpassing the residents and communicating directly with the attending physician could adversely affect rapport with medical resident colleagues. Likewise, communicating with them at an inopportune time, such as in the middle of their patient presentation and in front of the team, could also damage rapport. Additionally, pharmacy residents should realize that interactions may vary based on the setting. For example, in a community hospital, pharmacy residents may interact exclusively with preceptors and attending physicians. Likewise, this may occur in an ambulatory care setting, particularly when medical residents are not present. In the community setting, it may only occur one-to-one with a physician. When in doubt, always seek the advice of the pharmacist preceptor about effective communication styles.

> When in doubt, always seek the advice of the pharmacist preceptor about effective communication styles.

FUNCTIONING AS A MEMBER OF A TEAM

The pharmacist is a valuable member of the medical team who has an extremely important job. Knowing, understanding, and embracing that role are imperative to the success of the clinical pharmacist.

In order for patients to receive optimal medical care, members of the team must work together. Each member must execute his or her assignment every time in order for the team to be effective. As a pharmacy resident, the most damaging action that could occur is to fail to execute an assignment. Traits like tardiness, apathy, and laziness will prevent execution of assignments. Pharmacy residents should always arrive at the site early with a clear understanding of the preparatory work that needs to be completed. Residents must take personal responsibility for their actions; preparation is the resident's responsibility. Follow-up with preceptors or attending physicians if instructions are not completely clear. Failure to do so is a poor reflection on the resident, the residency program, and the profession of pharmacy.

> Pharmacy residents should always arrive at the site early with a clear understanding of the preparatory work that needs to be completed.

• The Patient As a Member of the Team

When considering all the members of the team, one should not neglect the most important party: the patient. Too often, professionals strive to provide the best care but neglect the patient's desires. Care plans should take into consideration the needs and wants of the patient. Do not forget that patients are individuals with cares, hopes, and feelings, and in the end, even the best plan must be implemented for it to be effective. When developing plans, there are multiple factors to be considered, including issues with adherence, cost, evidence for effectiveness, adverse effects, and the wishes and desires of the patient. Keeping this in mind, as well as any regional, cultural, generational, or ethnic factors, will aid one in designing a plan that is acceptable to all parties, including the patient.[5]

ADVICE FOR SUCCESS

Some universal etiquette should be considered a standard method of operation for any resident. Good hygiene is important as well as professional and neat attire. It is difficult to establish trust with patients and other professionals if the resident addresses them with unkempt hair, a shirt hanging out, and clothes that are noticeably wrinkled, even though the resident may have a wealth of knowledge to impart.[4] What constitutes professional dress can be debated, but suffice it to say that certain clothing is inappropriate to wear in the clinical setting. For example, cargo pants should never be substituted for dress slacks, and skirt hems should be visible from underneath the bottom of the lab coat. Women should avoid low-cut blouses or shirts. Neckties for males may be discouraged on some rotation sites for infection control issues, but in general, they are considered professional attire.

Always be humble, as pride commonly comes before destruction. Treat all healthcare workers as colleagues and with great respect, and remember that both colleagues and patients are people with hopes, cares, and fears. Deliver thoroughly researched, evidence-based recommendations in a collegial fashion, and always be well prepared for rounds, knowing patients as well as or better than the individual primarily responsible for their care. Do not become frustrated when a recommendation or care plan is not implemented, and learn from mentors what types of issues are worth discussing more vigorously.

> Deliver thoroughly researched, evidence-based recommendations in a collegial fashion.

THE FUTURE OF PHARMACIST-PROVIDED CARE

Had one asked the clinical pioneers of the 1960s if they would have pictured the profession in its current role, would they have expected less or more of us? As pharmacy education has evolved over the past 30 years, pharmacists are better equipped than ever to move from behind the counter to the bedside, but what does the future of our profession hold? Is consultant status and medication therapy management services the zenith of our profession, or is there something even better to come? Will some pharmacists one day provide a level of care more like a primary care provider to their patients? (A minority of pharmacists in a handful of states are already doing this.) These and many other questions are yet to be answered, because the answers to the questions lie within us. What we once were is no longer who we are now, and who we will be is not who we are now. One crucial question pertains to where we will go: will we wander aimlessly and allow other professions to dictate our status in the provision of healthcare? It is difficult to reach a destination when we don't know what that destination is. Hence, this challenge is issued: be responsible and professional while conducting duties, all the while focusing on the bright future and specific destinations the profession holds.

KEY POINTS

• Strive to provide evidence-based, patient-centered care that focuses on outcomes.

• Be prepared to provide a wide array of services in a variety of clinical settings.

• Always treat patients respectfully, following the golden rule.

• Demonstrate professionalism by being punctual, communicating effectively, understanding expectations, adhering to ethics, and acting with integrity.

• Do not settle for a suboptimal role as a practitioner; continue to promote the profession and be involved in a movement to continually transform pharmacy.

REFERENCES

1. Hibgy GJ. Pharmacy in the American century. *Pharm Times*. 1997;63:16–24.
2. American Association of Colleges of Pharmacy. Oath of a pharmacist. http://www.aacp.org/resources/academicpolicies/studentaffairspolicies/Documents/OATHOFAPHARMACIST2008–09.pdf. Accessed March 31, 2011.
3. American Pharmacists Association. White paper on pharmacy student professionalism. *J Am Pharm Assoc*. 2000;40:96–102.
4. Kahn MW. Etiquette-based medicine. *N Engl J Med*. 2008;358:1988–1989.
5. Stewart M, Brown JB, Donner A, et al. The impact of patient-centered care on outcomes. *J Fam Pract*. 2000;49:796–804.

CHAPTER 21

Teaching Responsibilities

Philip T. Rodgers and Jeffrey M. Tingen

Knowledge exists to be imparted.

—**Ralph Waldo Emerson**

....

QUESTIONS TO PONDER

1. What kind of didactic lecture methods are effective for residents to use to teach students?

2. What types of experiential teaching opportunities are available during a residency?

3. What is the purpose and value of teaching certificate programs offered by residency programs?

4. Is there a mentor in the program who could assist in the development of teaching abilities and styles?

5. What level of teaching is desired after completion of a residency?

....

Many pharmacy residents develop some desire to formally teach in their career, aspiring to be anything from an occasional preceptor to a tenure-track faculty member within a college or school of pharmacy.[1] Because of this widespread interest, pharmacy residency programs offer a variety of experiences in instructional techniques. The American Society of Health-System Pharmacists (ASHP) residency standards do not require accredited postgraduate year one (PGY1) programs to include formal teaching experiences, though it does provide goals and objectives for which PGY1 residents should be evaluated, depending on the situation (**Table 21-1**).

> ### Table 21-1 ASHP Outcome, Goal, and Objectives Related to Teaching for PGY1 Pharmacy Residency Programs
>
> *Outcome R5: Provide medication and practice-related education/training.*
>
> Goal R5.1: Provide effective medication and practice-related education, training, or counseling to patients, caregivers, healthcare professionals, and the public.
>
> - Objective R5.1.1: Use effective educational techniques in the design of all educational activities.
>
> - Objective R5.1.2: Design an assessment strategy that appropriately measures the specified objectives for education or training and fits the learning situation.
>
> - Objective R5.1.3: Use skill in the four preceptor roles employed in practice-based teaching (direct instruction, modeling, coaching, and facilitation).
>
> - Objective R5.1.4: Use skill in case-based teaching.
>
> - Objective R5.1.5: Use public speaking skills to speak effectively in large and small group situations.
>
> - Objective R5.1.6: Use knowledge of audiovisual aids and handouts to enhance the effectiveness of communications.
>
> *Source*: Adapted from American Society of Health-System Pharmacists. Required and elective outcomes, goals, objectives, and instructional objectives for postgraduate year one (PGY1) pharmacy residency programs, 2nd edition —effective July 2008. http://www.ashp.org/DocLibrary/Accreditation/PGY1-Goals-Objectives.aspx. Accessed March 31, 2011. Reprinted with permission.

This chapter focuses on formal teaching that may be included in a residency program, which is beyond teaching related to patient education that all pharmacists provide. It will consider the value of these experiences and their relationship to different levels of academia.

FORMAL TEACHING OPPORTUNITIES

The amount and types of teaching experiences available in residency programs vary. One program may offer little more than the opportunity to lead discussions with learners on rotation, and another may offer opportunities in direct preceptorship, didactic lectures, course coordination, and completion of a teaching certificate (**Table 21-2**).

The first essential question residents should ask themselves is if they want to participate in the formal education of students. If the answer is yes, then they should ask themselves what kind of formal teaching they want to do, and how much. Answering the first question is easy for some, but for others it may take the entire year to answer. Teaching is a great privilege and responsibility in the pharmacy profession. Pharmacists are expected to be experts in drug knowledge and to be lifelong learners. How can a student pharmacist become either of these without the help of excellent teachers? Pharmacists completing residency programs are exceptionally prepared with

> *Teaching is a great privilege and responsibility in the pharmacy profession.*

Table 21-2 Formal Teaching Opportunities for Pharmacy Residents

- Participating in or leading topic discussions with rotation students
- Discussing patient evaluations with students
- Teaching students from other professions (medical, nursing, etc.)
- In-service educational sessions
- Serving as a direct preceptor for a student pharmacist(s) on rotation
- Didactic lecture in a course at a college or school of pharmacy or other professional school
- Completion of a teaching certificate
- Continuing education programs
- Journal club or case conference
- Teaching assistant in a pharmacy skills lab
- Assisting with course coordination at a college or school of pharmacy or other school
- Participation with a school-based committee related to curriculum

clinical knowledge to impart to learners someday. Some may even consider it an obligation to teach those who come later as a way to give back to the profession.

When a resident decides to seek teaching opportunities, it is wise to seek a teaching mentor or advisor. This person could be the residency program director (RPD), a close preceptor, or a faculty member with a local college or school of pharmacy. Likely, it will be a teacher whose instructional style the resident hopes to emulate. This mentor may also assist with the initial building of a teaching portfolio and familiarize the resident with academic faculty systems.

To develop as an effective teacher, the resident also needs specific feedback on his or her teaching techniques, and this may not be the expertise of the primary preceptors and clinicians with whom the resident is working. The faculty mentor could assist by providing critical feedback in a timely manner about the effectiveness of the teaching methods used by the resident, help the resident explore new teaching methods, and assist the resident in evaluation of learners. The resident should also seek feedback from his or her students. Although this feedback could be skewed due to the difficulty of the material or other the circumstances beyond the resident's control, any student feedback should be discussed with the mentor to help the resident grow.

Effective teaching also requires excellent communication skills for both one-on-one teaching and public speaking. It requires confident knowledge and application of various advanced instructional techniques, such as case-based or problem-based instruction or clinical (bedside) teaching. It requires insight into appropriate critical evaluation approaches and the ability to provide valuable feedback to the learner. Effective teaching also requires patience and empathy to assist the student throughout the process, rather than doing it for the learner.

The extent of formal teaching a resident wishes to undertake in his or her career may dictate the amount of residency training to pursue. To serve as a preceptor, often a PGY1 residency will be adequate, and becoming a clinical faculty member within a college or school of pharmacy will sometimes require completion of a postgraduate year two (PGY2) specialty. In the end, teaching can be an extremely rewarding endeavor in a professional career.

TEACHING CERTIFICATES: COMPONENTS AND VALUE

Teaching certificate programs are important features of many PGY1 and PGY2 pharmacy residencies. However, at this time, there is no standard for the learning goals of a teaching certificate from ASHP or other pharmacy organizations. Teaching certificate programs are designed to teach residents how to teach in order to further their residency training experience and to allow residents to develop teaching skills that will be useful in many aspects of the pharmacy profession.[2] Residents who complete teaching certificate programs may choose to pursue a career in academia, although not all residents may have the desire to engage in student pharmacist development in an academic setting. A teaching certificate may be beneficial for other modes of teaching, as well.

Most teaching certificate programs share a similar foundation upon which they are based, but each program will have its own specific characteristics. A teaching certificate program is a goal-oriented curriculum that allows the resident to work toward specific requirements. Teaching certificate programs generally require the resident to attend formal seminars in which pertinent teaching topics are covered. The number of seminars that each teaching certificate program offers varies widely. With the growth of residency programs that are not in close proximity with one another, some teaching certificate programs have moved toward utilization of distance education, providing sessions through web-based learning modules with limited face-to-face seminars. Residents are generally required to attend all sessions in order to complete the program.

A teaching certificate program is a goal-oriented curriculum that allows the resident to work toward specific requirements.

Seminars are normally developed and taught by experienced pharmacy faculty members, but they are not limited to this set of professionals. RPDs are often members of seminar faculty if they have a large teaching role within the academic institution. Other possible seminar leaders may include faculty affiliated with the university's school of education, and these outside faculty members may present topics related to the foundation of education and education strategies that may be useful in the classroom setting. Examples of teaching certificate program seminars are listed in **Table 21-3**.

Table 21-3 Examples of Teaching Certificate Program Seminars

- Basics of education
- Technology in the classroom
- Course planning
- Enhancement of student-centered learning
- Student assessment
- Professionalism and civility in the classroom
- Preceptorship
- Student and faculty assessments

Teaching certificate programs also have one vital component in addition to attendance of scheduled seminars: teaching. Residents may be responsible for providing didactic lectures in addition to precepting students as part of teaching certificate requirements. Examples of lectures may include conducting a formal didactic lecture at the university or leading small-group discussions throughout the semester in a particular course. In addition, student pharmacist precepting responsibilities may also be part of the teaching certificate program. The resident will normally serve as a copreceptor, or possibly the primary preceptor, for student pharmacists and will be responsible for discussions, projects, and evaluations of the student during the designated period. Precepting is often challenging for the pharmacy resident, and teaching certificate programs assist in developing the skills that are needed to become an effective preceptor.

Many teaching certificate programs encourage or require pharmacy residents to develop a teaching portfolio. Teaching portfolios should include three key components: personal statement of teaching, overview of teaching accomplishments and activities, and verification of successful activities through feedback from colleagues and students.[3] Teaching portfolios are not limited to formal didactic lectures; they can also include any educational presentation for an audience.

Most individuals consider the personal statement of teaching to be the most difficult portion of the teaching portfolio. It is a personal reflection of the principles that make a great educator and the impact the writer plans to have as an educator. Although these statements are personal and customized to the individual, common areas to address include purpose for teaching, approach to teaching in the classroom and on advanced pharmacy practice experiences and goals for self-development of teaching skills. Building a teaching portfolio during residency training will provide the groundwork for professional accomplishments in the forthcoming pharmacy career.[4]

The value of a teaching certificate program is immense. Many pharmacy educators today did not have the opportunity to complete formal training. Regardless of whether or not the resident wants to pursue a career in academia, teaching certificate programs provide the opportunity to develop skills that can be utilized in any practice setting.[3] Teaching certificate programs afford us great appreciation for our pharmacy educators and are an asset to any pharmacy residency training program.[4]

EXPERIENTIAL TEACHING ROLES BY RESIDENTS

Precepting is one of the most satisfying roles that pharmacy residents can undertake.

Experiential education is an important part of development and training of student pharmacists during their pharmacy education. Experiential education is conducted by faculty members, pharmacist preceptors, and occasionally other healthcare professionals. During residency training, residents may be expected to serve in a preceptor role for student pharmacists. Precepting is one of the most satisfying roles that pharmacy residents can undertake during residency training.

As a preceptor, the resident may serve as the main individual responsible for the student learner. The pharmacy resident may be responsible for advanced pharmacy practice experience (APPE) coordination, including creation of student schedules, assignment of student projects, evaluation of student presentations, and evaluation of student progress during the APPE. In addition, depending on the residency program, a pharmacy resident may be on a rotation experience with student pharmacists. When this occurs, the pharmacy resident may not serve as the primary preceptor but may serve in a supervisory capacity as copreceptor, since the pharmacy resident is a more advanced learner than student pharmacists are.

Precepting by pharmacy residents also presents many challenges. Occasionally, pharmacy residents may precept students they know on a personal level if their residency program is affiliated with their alma mater. Even if this is not the case, the pharmacy resident is a fresh new practitioner not far removed from pharmacy school rotations. It is sometimes difficult for pharmacy residents to establish boundaries and ground rules with student pharmacists because pharmacy residents identify closely with student pharmacists. In order to avoid problems with establishing boundaries with students, it is extremely important for the pharmacy resident to be professional, respectful, and organized. If a pharmacy resident is having difficulty establishing a role as a preceptor, the resident should consult with his or her preceptor, RPD, or other mentors to obtain situation-specific advice about how to better handle the precepting role.

Depending on the residency program practice setting, the pharmacy resident may participate in experiential teaching for other healthcare professional students or learners. Academic medical centers and other practice sites host a number of students, such as medical, nursing, physical therapy, physician assistant, and other allied health students, as well as healthcare professional graduate students, such as medical residents. These students often seek out pharmacy residents because they are accessible, approachable, and share a common bond as young practitioners. Although pharmacy residents are rarely responsible for teaching other healthcare professional students, this opportunity, when available, can provide an enriching experience that mimics real-world education provided by pharmacists to other healthcare professionals.

The ability to effectively evaluate learners on rotation is a common area of consternation by preceptors. Quality evaluations include both positive feedback and constructive criticism in a balanced, unbiased, and nonpersonal manner, and they help students engage in their own self-evaluation. Designing and conducting a good evaluation is a learned process for most preceptors and residents, but it is critical. Pharmacy residents should consult their RPD and other preceptors to identify best practices for experiential teaching and evaluation. Furthermore, most teaching certificate programs attempt to incorporate seminars on experiential teaching and evaluation into the curriculum for residents. Seasoned practitioners often provide excellent insight into establishing pharmacy resident credibility with student learners and assist in how to deal with struggling or confrontational student learners.[5] Becoming an effective preceptor is an acquired skill and rarely comes naturally to new practitioners. Opportunities to participate in experiential education during residency training offers pharmacy residents yet another opportunity to enhance their skill set in order to become effective pharmacist practitioners and educators of student pharmacists, pharmacist peers, and other healthcare providers.

DIDACTIC TEACHING OPPORTUNITIES

The opportunities for a resident to provide didactic teaching may be limited, depending on what affiliation the residency institution has with academic institutions such as colleges or schools of pharmacy, nursing, medicine, or others. According to one study, just over half of PGY1 residents (57%) gave a lecture at a school during residency, and just under half (48%) also taught a seminar course as a teaching experience. The percentage was higher for programs associated with a college

Residents who aspire to faculty positions should actively seek opportunities to teach at a college or school.

or school of pharmacy and for those residents who took a faculty position after residency.[6] Residents who aspire to faculty positions should actively seek opportunities to teach at a college or school near their residency. For programs affiliated with a college or school of pharmacy, this is easy to do. For programs independent of a college or school of pharmacy, the resident will have to seek opportunities from preceptors who may be adjunct faculty or instructors at healthcare professional schools, including nonpharmacy programs, such as nursing, allied health, or medicine.

Teaching to a classroom full of students is often a stress-inducing event for a resident, requiring hours of preparation and worry. How can a resident ensure excellence in this experience? Several preparatory steps will help. As noted previously, the supervision of a faculty mentor or advisor is important for getting feedback. Upon assignment of a topic for a class, the resident should understand the background of the students involved because there is a significant difference among teaching methods for first-year and third-year student pharmacists. Know how large of a class it will be. Dynamic, participatory lectures may be limited in a classroom of 30 students or more, and a class of more than 100 students may be downright intimidating to a new resident.

The next thing to understand is the course. Is there a set format for lectures? Some classes may have rules about how to use slides, cases, problem-based learning, and/or audience-response systems. The resident should make sure he or she has the resources to create these materials. For example, is a special program necessary for an audience-response system? The resident may be able to get materials used in previous years and modify them to meet his or her needs. However, residents should not rely solely on older material because updates to information will likely be needed, and residents should present the material in their own style so they can be more familiar with it. If the course coordinator does not particularly restrict teaching styles, the resident should decide with a mentor what teaching method would work best, in light of what areas of growth the resident wants to develop. In general, most schools appreciate instructors going beyond one-way didactic lectures and encourage class participation and problem solving. Thus, the resident will want to explore methods to bring patient cases or theoretical problems before the class for discussion.

The first and most important step in designing a lecture or activity is to create or revise learning objectives in order to delineate the road map for where the activity will go. Materials, such as slides or cases, should be developed in light of these objectives. During the learning session, the resident should be prepared for diversions generated by questions from students. Practicing lecture-based portions of the class will help the resident stay on track.

The resident will often be asked to develop test questions for the topic being taught. The resident should work closely with a mentor to write effective questions, whether they are multiple choice, short answer, patient note writing, true–false, or complex K-type questions. This process can be quite challenging, and the resident should seek references that assist with high-quality test question writing. The mentor's advice can be a valuable asset in evaluating the quality of questions and suggesting improvements for better questions.

KEY POINTS

+ Residency programs offer many opportunities for residents to work in a variety of teaching environments and use numerous styles; these activities help determine whether to pursue a teaching career.

+ Residents should explore a variety of didactic classroom teaching techniques to expand their teaching experiences beyond basic lectures, such as case presentations, problem solving, and audience participation.

- Residents play an integral part in student pharmacists' experiential education, as well as that of pharmacists and other healthcare professionals.

- Teaching certificate programs provide opportunities for residents to gain formal training in effective teaching skills that can be utilized in all practice settings.

- A teaching mentor can provide direction regarding teaching effectiveness and evaluative feedback of students.

REFERENCES

1. Smith KM, Romanelli F. Use of an electronic survey to assess the training and practice experiences of pharmacy residency graduates. *Am J Health Syst Pharm.* 2005;62:2283–2288.
2. Romanelli F, Smith KM, Brandt BF. Teaching residents how to teach: a scholarship of teaching and learning certificate programs (STLC) for pharmacy residents. *Am J Pharm Educ.* 2005;69:126–132.
3. Johnson PN, Smith K. The teaching portfolio: a useful guide for pharmacists' teaching goals. *Am J Health Syst Pharm.* 2007;64:352–365.
4. Castellani V, Haber SL, Ellis SC. Evaluation of teaching certificate programs for pharmacy residents. *Am J Health Syst Pharm.* 2003;60:1037–1041.
5. Carr LS. Teaching as a new practitioner. *Am J Health Syst Pharm.* 2006;63:1400–1404.
6. McNatty D, Cox C, Seifert CF. Assessment of teaching experiences completed during accredited pharmacy residency programs. *Am J Pharm Educ.* 2007;71:88.

CHAPTER 22

Scholarship Responsibilities

Kelly M. Smith

Build a better mousetrap and the world will beat a path to your door.

—**Ralph Waldo Emerson**

QUESTIONS TO PONDER

1. How does scholarship differ from research?
2. How can scholarship be achieved in a practice setting?
3. What skills are needed to conduct pharmacy scholarship?
4. Where can one find resources for scholarship development?
5. Why is scholarship an important feature of residency training?

According to the American Society of Health-System Pharmacists (ASHP) residency accreditation standards, residents are required to demonstrate project management skills. Such skill development may take the form of formal research, continuous quality improvement initiatives, medication use evaluations, or practice service implementation (e.g., protocol implementation with measurement of impact, or quality assurance initiatives) that benefit the host organization. Residents can readily transform these efforts into scholarship. In addition to residency projects, some programs may give residents other scholarly opportunities such as publishing review articles and/or book chapters. Although these are important types of scholarship, this chapter focuses on residency projects with dissemination of findings via poster, presentation, or publication.

SCHOLARSHIP DEFINED

Scholarship is commonly defined as the creation, discovery, advancement, or transformation of knowledge.[1] It exceeds the conduct of research because simply discovering information without disseminating it to others for critical evaluation holds little meaning. To transform a process from project management or research (i.e., answering a scientific question) to scholarship, one must display elements of originality, creativity, peer review, and communication. These extra steps benefit not only the individual or institution in which the investigation was conducted, but also the profession and patients beyond the immediate practice setting.

Advancing the practice of pharmacy is fully reliant upon scholarship, whether it is therapeutics, optimal use of technology, medication safety, assessing the role of the pharmacist in patient care delivery, or conducting new approaches to pharmacy education and training. A practice-based investigation is the most common currency of scholarship for a pharmacy practitioner. One does not need to conduct a clinical trial comparing the effects of an emerging therapy with a gold standard treatment to be considered a scholar. Scholarship may include identifying an issue of importance in healthcare (e.g., a rapid increase of prolonged hospital stays due to undesired responses to warfarin reversal), attacking the issue (e.g., creation and evaluation of a new vitamin K dosing protocol), and then disseminating the results (e.g., presenting a poster at a national pharmacy meeting). These activities may meet a local need for the hospital, and they may also provide strategies for external clinicians who face similar clinical dilemmas.

> A practice-based investigation is the most common currency of scholarship for a pharmacy practitioner.

THE SCHOLAR'S TOOL KIT

Conducting scholarship is not dependent on a formal faculty appointment, extensive research training, or large-scale grant funding. However, it is reliant on a number of skills, attitudes, and approaches. Scholarship can take the form of discovery, application, integration, or teaching.[1] Keep in mind that scholarship may also be performed as an assessment of unique patient responses to therapy (i.e., case report), an approach to addressing a dilemma encountered while managing a pharmacy department, or other observational report.

• Spirit of Inquiry

A desire to fully understand a process, response to therapy, or phenomenon in practice may be the most important attitude for a successful scholar. Both yearning to know why and then setting about to answer the question provides the fuel to power any investigation.

• Creating a Plan

Undertaking any project or inquiry, even if it is not anticipated to be taken to the level of scholarship, requires an orderly, planned approach to be successful. Mining the existing literature determines if there is a gap in evidence, which not only helps avoid repeating the work of others, but also reveals others' approaches and setbacks so that history is not repeated.

• Defining the Question

Considering limited resources and time during the residency year, the resident must distill an inquiry to a discrete, measurable question or task. Otherwise, the endpoint may never be reached. For instance, setting about to measure the effects of a pharmacist-provided diabetes management service can entail a number of variables, confounders, and other elements that influence the findings. Focusing on one specific value that reflects the impact of the service on patient care (e.g., mean change in HbA1c over six months) will likely yield a better assessment of the program's impact. When the question has been determined, narrow the scope of investigation further by using the acronym PICO (patients, intervention, comparison, outcomes) (**Table 22-1**).[2]

• Gaining Support

Many projects will require review and approval by the local institutional review board. This requirement will vary among institutions, even for quality improvement or practice-based research.[3] Other site-specific committees may need to be consulted for approval. For instance, Veterans Affairs sites have their own internal research approval processes. Beyond gaining approval for the project, seek the input of colleagues with experience in the field because they may be able to identify additional elements to consider. There may also be an opportunity to gain extramural (external) funding to underwrite the costs of conducting the investigation. This approach is commonly referred to as grantsmanship, involving a competitive process to petition for funds based on proposed scientific merit and budgetary measures.

Table 22-1 Factors That Shape Project Design (PICO)

Patients: Which population (or data set) will be evaluated?

Intervention: How will the impact of a new process be measured? What other elements may affect the results?

Comparison: Should there be a comparison against another group, other baseline data, or some other measure?

Outcomes: What are the specific, measurable end points that will be used to answer the question?

Source: Adapted from Smith KM. Building upon existing evidence to shape future research endeavors. *Am J Health Syst Pharm*. 2008;65:1767–1774.

• Conducting the Investigation

Project success will most likely result from an organized, detailed approach, with timelines set for each element.

A number of approaches can be pursued to gather a sufficient amount of data to answer an investigative question. Project success will most likely result from an organized, detailed approach, with timelines set for each element. It is important to ensure that the data collection tools allow for the capture of information needed for analysis. Following data collection, analysis and assessment must occur so that the resident can assemble an answer to the research question.

• Disseminating the Results

Sharing results with others and benefitting from their critical analysis through peer review are essential features of scholarship.

Upon the conclusion of an investigation, it may be difficult for the resident to maintain enthusiasm for the next step: preparing an abstract for poster or podium presentation at a professional meeting or assembling a manuscript for submission to a biomedical journal. Yet, sharing results with others and benefitting from their critical analysis through peer review are essential features of scholarship. Considering the countless hours that were devoted to the project, failing to close the loop on the process by not pursuing publication or presentation would be letting oneself down.

Identifying a suitable venue to present the project's results can be challenging for some residents.[4] However, reviewing past issues of a journal and abstracts of previous meeting presentations can provide insight into the types of projects or topics that may be consistent with the venue's focus. Many pharmacy residents present their project results at one of the seven resident conferences that occur annually, including Eastern States, Great Lakes, Midwest, Midsouth, Southeast, Southwest Leadership, and Western States.[5] The physical location of the residency program determines which conference residents attend. Local or state pharmacy society meetings may also offer poster or pearl presentations, affording the resident an opportunity to learn the presentation process in this type of venue. Those same groups often publish newsletters or journals that provide excellent opportunities for publication of practice-based research.

The ASHP Foundation commissioned a series of articles, published in the *American Journal of Health-System Pharmacy*, designed to assist pharmacy practitioners in conducting practice-based research.[6] Residents are encouraged to view these articles, as well as other resources, on the foundation's website.

PROJECT TIMELINE

The adage "failing to plan is planning to fail" certainly holds true for a resident project, given the finite duration of a residency. Several rate-limiting steps must be considered to ensure the project is completed by the end of the residency year. Although there is no timeline that will work for every investigation, some key steps should be considered. The plan for the project should be assembled and reviewed by preceptors and other collaborators before data is collected. Thus, settling on a well-defined focus for the inquiry and determining the project methods must be completed early in the residency year, as early as September. The resident may need to obtain additional training in human subject research in order to be eligible to complete the project. This step, too, must be completed early in the process. Completing data collection by December or January is an admirable goal because it allows for data analysis in the early winter months and produces sufficient results for presentation at regional residency conferences in the spring. Submission of the project for a podium or poster presentation and preparing the final project manuscript can then culminate with the conclusion of the residency year. Residents are referred to other sources that provide numerous tools to support these important steps in the scholarship process.[7-9]

KEY POINTS

- Residents can elevate research to scholarship by sharing the results of a formal investigation and improving the presentation of that information based on peer review.

- Practice-based investigations are as meaningful as original clinical research or discoveries of new molecular entities.

- A structured, organized approach to an investigation that is shaped by existing evidence is recommended for a successful project.

- Residency training affords residents the time to develop scholarly abilities under the guidance of and with support from seasoned colleagues.

- ASHP has developed a number of practitioner-focused resources that support the development of both research and scholarship skills.

REFERENCES

1. Boyer EL. *Scholarship Reconsidered: Priorities of the Professoriate*. Princeton, NJ: The Carnegie Foundation for the Advancement of Teaching; 1990.
2. Smith KM. Building upon existing evidence to shape future research endeavors. *Am J Health Syst Pharm*. 2008;65:1767–1774.
3. Johnson N, Vermeulen L, Smith KM. A survey of academic medical centers to distinguish between quality improvement and research activities. *Q Manage Health Care*. 2006;15:215–220.
4. Vazquez SR. Publishing your residency project. *Am J Health Syst Pharm*. 2010;67:1058–1059.
5. American Society of Health-System Pharmacists. Reasons to complete a residency. http://www.ashp.org/menu/Residents/PGY1/WhyaResidency.aspx Accessed May 31, 2011.
6. ASHP Foundation. Research fundamentals. http://www.ashpfoundation.org/ MainMenuCategories/ResearchResourceCenter/FosteringYoungInvestigators/ AJHPResearchFundamentalsSeries.aspx. Accessed March 31, 2011.

7. Kane-Gill S, Olsen KM. How to write an abstract suitable for publication. *Hosp Pharm.* 2004;39:289–292.

8. Miller JE. Preparing and presenting effective research posters. *Health Serv Res.* 2007;42:311–328.

9. Welch HG. Preparing manuscripts for submission to medical journals: the paper trail. *Eff Clin Pract.* 1999;2:131–137.

CHAPTER 23

What's Next? Options After Residency Training

John B. Bossaer and Michael A. Decoske

Luck is what happens when preparation meets opportunity.

—**Seneca**

QUESTIONS TO PONDER

1. What are the strengths and weaknesses of the resident?
2. What are 5-, 10-, and 15-year career goals?
3. How can a resident achieve his or her goals?
4. How does a clinician stay current on professional and scientific research?
5. What can the future pharmacist do to give back to the profession?

When a pharmacy resident approaches completion of the residency program, it is undoubtedly an exciting and nerve-racking time. A residency certificate represents countless hours of hard work, long days, short nights, and a passion for professional development. Now it is time to reflect on the skills developed during the residency and to look ahead into the pharmacist's professional future. This chapter addresses the multiple options after residency training.

SWOT ANALYSIS

Complete the SWOT analysis by realistically and honestly assessing professional and personal strengths, weaknesses, opportunities, and threats.

Residents should take a brief moment to perform an internal personal *SWOT* (strengths, weakness, opportunities, threats) analysis as they contemplate the next step after completing the residency program.[1] This simple exercise will help to organize planning and allow for a better understanding of one's professional self before embarking on future career steps. Consider the strengths and areas to improve that were identified during the residency search (see Chapter 13, "The Application Process," and Chapter 14, "The On-Site Interview") and at the start of the residency (see Chapter 18, "Developing a Personal Mission and Leadership Style"). Complete the SWOT analysis by realistically and honestly assessing professional and personal strengths, weaknesses, opportunities, and threats (**Figure 23-1**).

Strengths	Weaknesses
Opportunities	**Threats**

Figure 23-1: SWOT Analysis to Assess Professional and Personal Strengths, Weaknesses, Opportunities, and Threats

• **Strengths**

What are the core strengths the resident developed as a pharmacist? Having completed a residency, a practitioner can rest assured that his or her clinical skills are strong and varied. What clinical areas are most enticing? Which patient population motivated the resident to put forth his or her best? Perhaps the resident particularly excelled in some other areas of the residency program such as research, publications, or public speaking. Was the resident particularly motivated by opportunities to participate in medication therapy management, to teach and precept students, to perform drug use evaluations, or to find ways that the hospital could improve efficiency and save money? There is a good chance that these strengths represent a resident's passion, and they provide avenues to seek opportunities that can make use of these strengths in the future.

• **Weaknesses**

What are a resident's weaknesses as a pharmacist? Now is not the time to use the interview trick of subtly turning a weakness into a strength. Assess weaknesses honestly. Although the resident is likely more confident than he or she was upon graduation of pharmacy school, is self-confidence a concern? On the other hand, did the resident have a reputation as a know-it-all (or someone who thinks he or she knows it all)? Conversely, did the resident have a difficult time making decisions, always second guessing or trying to perfect every detail? Maybe the resident struggled to stay current with literature or had trouble conducting independent scholarship. Are there a few nagging areas of practice that feel foreign or uncomfortable and that, for one reason or another, never really sunk in? If an applicant is unsure of the weaknesses that are most important, ask what weakness may prevent an employer from offering a position. Some employers may be interested in hiring only pharmacists with postgraduate year two (PGY2) training or those with board certification. When a weakness is identified, a plan for improvement can be incorporated into a personal professional development plan.

• **Opportunities and Threats**

It is beneficial to take time to evaluate the opportunities and threats to career advancement. Following a residency, opportunities can be limitless; however, pharmacists should be realistic and carefully think through what opportunities exist as a result of residency training, as well as his or her financial and personal circumstances. In addition, there is value in tempering the opportunities with potential threats. How many pharmacists entering the job market have similar skills? There are far more pharmacists with postgraduate year one (PGY1) training than PGY2 training, so a PGY1-trained pharmacist looking for a clinical specialist or faculty position may be competing against a more qualified applicant pool. Consider that as a potential threat. Additionally, is the goal to find a dream job in a dream city? Many colleagues share that dream.

YOUR VISION, YOUR FUTURE

No one cares more about your career future than you.

Remember this simple truth: no one cares more about your career future than you. Now, consider that dream job. Are any of the following elements, or others like them, part of the vision?

- Wearing scrubs in the ER while running a code

- Lecturing in front of pharmacy or medical students

- Wearing a white coat and counseling patients prior to hospital discharge

- Providing pharmacokinetic services at a rural hospital

- Helping to establish medication policy for an entire hospital as a clinical coordinator

- Participating in managed care formulary decisions that will directly affect thousands of covered lives for a particular healthcare plan

- Running a pharmacotherapy clinic

- Traveling the world in the pharmaceutical industry

- Presenting innovative research or expertise at a national meeting

- Expanding clinical pharmacy services within a chain of community pharmacies

- Poring over data to determine the cost-effectiveness of a particular therapy for a given population of patients

There is, of course, no wrong answer. In fact, unlimited dream jobs exist, but the road to each varies. To be sure, there are multiple roads to the same position, and one road may be better suited for one person than another. Preparing for what course a career may take ahead of time will give the resident the best chance to make the most of every career opportunity, whether it is an internal promotion or accepting a new and exciting position elsewhere.

• Realistic First Job Expectations

It may not be realistic to expect the first job out of residency training to be a dream job.

It may not be realistic to expect the first job out of residency training to be a dream job. Just as a head coach must first work as an assistant coach, pharmacists also must gain experience and, to one extent or another, pay their dues before climbing the employment ladder. A clinical coordinator of a large academic medical center hospital may not be able to perform successfully his or her job without first excelling as a clinical pharmacist. Likewise, it would not be prudent to start a consulting pharmacy business without first building the skills and resume as a clinician or subject matter expert.

A first job out of residency will likely be very different from the position of a resident. The new practitioner is now the go-to person, responsible for decisions without the luxury of a scrutinizing preceptor. A resident may have been shielded from the full scope of participation in departmental initiatives, but a new practitioner can expect greater responsibility to serve on committees and to take the lead on quality improvement initiatives and medication use evaluations. Invariably, new practitioners will encounter situations for which they do not feel adequately prepared. Moreover, new practitioners may find themselves doubting their skills and abilities. These feelings are not uncommon after moving on from residency, especially if the first job is outside the institution where one trained. New pharmacists should be diligent and trust in the skills and abilities gained during residency.

LIFELONG LEARNING BEGINS NOW

In addition to the change in responsibilities, the learning needs of a new practitioner change as well. Residents typically spend a great deal of time reviewing standards of therapy and catching up on years of pharmacotherapy that preceded their pharmacy career. This information is often new to the resident or learned in much more detail than before, with a strong emphasis on evidence-based medicine. As an independent new practitioner, the onus for staying current on such knowledge falls squarely on the individual because there is no longer a preceptor or program director to foster such learning. Daily electronic mailing lists and electronic tables of contents (eTOC) for selected medical journals serve as efficient and concise ways to stay current with pertinent medical literature. It can be helpful to take just 15 minutes upon arriving to work to scan these electronic mailing lists and eTOCs. Scanning the abstract may be sufficient for issues not pertinent to one's individual practice. However, potential landmark and practice-changing articles should be identified, printed out, and set aside for future in-depth critiquing. Sending information directly to an e-mail inbox instead of a pharmacist expending valuable time and energy to pull it can be extraordinarily helpful in keeping up to date. Set up a personal daily information infusion system and stick to it, tweaking it along the way. In addition, one cannot discount the lifelong learning provided by membership and participation in professional societies and annual meetings with quality continuing education programming. Implementing a continuous professional development routine is essential to taking the next step as a new practitioner.[1]

One important way to document continued learning is by becoming a Board Certified Pharmacotherapy Specialist (BCPS). Many individuals consider this option upon completion of residency training. To sit for the examination, a candidate must have a current pharmacy license and three

One important way to document continued learning is by becoming a Board Certified Pharmacotherapy Specialist (BCPS).

years of practice experience with at least 50% of the time in pharmacotherapy activities or the completion of a PGY1 residency. If a residency is used to establish eligibility for the examination, effective January 1, 2013, the residency must be accredited by the American Society of Health-System Pharmacists (ASHP) or another recognized body.

Residents continuing on to a PGY2 residency following successful completion of a PGY1 residency should consider sitting for the pharmacotherapy board certification exam. There are advantages and disadvantages to sitting for this exam in the fall of a PGY2 residency. A PGY2 residency requires a significant time commitment. Many PGY2 residents may find it difficult to manage the residency duties at a high level while preparing to take the board certification; however, PGY2 residents are often specializing in unique areas of practice. The board certification exam tests for knowledge on a wide variety of topics that many residents feel most comfortable and experienced with immediately following a PGY1 residency. Since this clinical knowledge is likely still fresh in the mind of a PGY2 resident, it may actually be the best time to take the test. Some residency programs may not have a budget to reimburse residents for the significant costs associated with the exam, but the pharmacy department of an employer may cover the cost for those who sit for and pass the board certification exam as an incentive for nonresident staff members.

There are numerous specialties beyond pharmacotherapy where certification can be obtained through the Board of Pharmacy Specialties, including ambulatory care, nuclear, nutrition support, oncology, and psychiatry, as well as added qualifications (e.g., infectious diseases, cardiology).[2] BCPS and other recognized certifications are an important way for new practitioners to begin to establish credibility in an area of practice.

While working to establish credibility with peers and healthcare professionals at a new practice, a new practitioner may feel tempted to jump at every opportunity that crosses his or her desk or in-box. This is an area where extreme caution is necessary. There is great temptation to say yes to every project or opportunity, but remember that no is not a bad word. New practitioners do not want to overextend themselves and risk burnout. Rather, one wants to be able complete the tasks assigned and deliver high-quality work. Obviously, required tasks from an employer would not fit into the no category, but optional assignments or opportunities may. Remember, a career is a marathon, not a sprint. One cannot transition from a first job to a dream job overnight. Carefully evaluate opportunities to take on added responsibility and select the ones that best suit the employer's needs and one's career aspirations. Take time and savor the opportunities that arise. Additionally, knowledge of personal and professional strengths and weaknesses will help identify opportunities that utilize one's unique skill set to its maximum level.

> Remember, a career is a marathon, not a sprint.

POSTRESIDENCY POSITIONS

Residency training will prepare graduates of the program for a wide variety of potential career options. These options will differ based on the type(s) of residency program(s) a new practitioner has completed.

• Clinical Pharmacist–Specialist

Most residency-trained pharmacists take positions as clinical pharmacists or clinical specialists. What is the difference? It will likely vary on the practice model of the institution. In general, clinical pharmacists provide a variety of integrated clinical pharmacy services to multiple patient populations, and a clinical specialist provides clinical pharmacy services of greater depth, knowledge, and skill within a specialty patient population, such as oncology or pediatrics. Other responsibilities vary by institution and practice model, such as order entry and review, sterile product or unit dose distribution, research, teaching opportunities, and committee work. Many current residents target a particular type of position because their residency preceptors practice in similar positions. Although these positions may be professionally satisfying, individuals should not discount consideration of other career options as well.

• Academia

Residents may pursue a career in academia, such as a clinical (or nontenure) track position within a college or school of pharmacy.[3] Responsibilities usually include teaching (both didactic and experiential), professional service (clinical practice), research, and service to the college or academic institution (serving on committees). The balance of these four pillars will vary based on a person's skills and desires and the needs of the institution. Most practitioners in clinical track positions spend the majority of their time in practice, but also spend time teaching in the classroom, on patient care rounds, in the clinic, or in topic discussions and journal clubs. Some positions may be entirely funded by the college, but many will be cofunded by the university and the practice site. Responsibilities for such positions must be carefully explored, and the expectations of both entities should be clearly articulated. Graduating residents must be careful to avoid split-funded positions that really require two full-time pharmacists. Although academia may offer less by way of starting salary compared to a clinical pharmacy position, many will find that the academic freedom and time to pursue scholarship and research are suitable trade-offs. The importance of understanding the entire compensation package cannot be overstated.

LOOKING FOR THE FIRST JOB

Weighing the pros and cons of a potential first position out of residency will no doubt parallel the decision-making process used in evaluating residency programs. One will consider location, livability, salary and benefits, prestige, and probably gut intuition. Additional consideration should also be given to opportunities for growth and professional development. An ideal first job will assist the pharmacist in his or her preparation for the dream job in a variety of ways. For example, a new practitioner may have an opportunity for promotion from clinical pharmacist to clinical manager or clinical coordinator. Consider if the position can offer additional experience or the opportunity to strengthen a professional weakness.

Given the advancement of pharmacy in recent years, many residents entertain the possibility of taking on newly created positions or starting new services. Such positions offer a great deal in the way of creativity and satisfaction. As the first person to hold the position, a new practitioner would have the opportunity to create the service from scratch and take pride in witnessing what may be a transformation in care. However, such an opportunity will come with unique challenges. The pharmacist would be required to traverse uncharted waters with clinicians who may not have experience with pharmacy services and may initially be wary of a perceived turf war. In addition, developing the clinical infrastructure, including policies and procedures, clinical protocols, intervention documentation, and billing may all need to be created from scratch. Before diving in to the process, find a mentor who has followed a similar course and is willing to share his or her experiences. Also, be sure to do a thorough literature review and to reach out through professional networks for advice and guidance.

TAKING THE NEXT STEP

Finding positions after residency is a little different from finding a residency program. The Personnel Placement Service (PPS) at ASHP's Midyear Clinical Meeting (MCM) is usually a great place to start; however, there is no clinical pharmacist showcase to locate positions. Organizations often advertise positions in several locations, depending on the position requirements.[4] In addition to the PPS at the MCM, the online listing of the American College of Clinical Pharmacy (ACCP) is another great place to search.[5] Many positions are discovered not through advertisement, but rather through word of mouth or networking. Building a strong network of professional contacts is made possible by being active in local, regional, and national professional organizations, committees and group projects, and leveraging the professional network of preceptors and residency program directors. Such a diverse network is a great place to learn about job opportunities as well as career advancement opportunities, including participation in continuing education workshops, presenting at national meetings, and involvement in research projects.

No matter where a resident would like to see his or her career go, the chances of successfully reaching that goal will increase by identifying good mentors.[6,7] A good mentor is willing to share life experiences, and holds, or has held, a position the new practitioner would like to hold one day. For example, if a new practitioner desires to be director of pharmacy, what better person to serve as a mentor than a current or past director of pharmacy? Such a mentor can provide real, practical guidance on what works and what to avoid. Consider having a few mentors, one a few years older on a similar career path and others who are more advanced. In any case, look for a mentor with similar professional qualities and values who instills confidence and trust.

Although networking and mentorship will no doubt be helpful in reaching career goals, one's ultimate career path must be self-directed. A dream job is likely a dream job for a reason: not just anyone can do it. This means new practitioners must work to develop themselves into experts in their given field. This process will not occur overnight; it takes continued development. Practitioners should find ways each day to enhance one's skills. After days upon days of incremental improvements, new practitioners may indeed find themselves transformed into a pharmacist who is ready for that dream job.

In the process of improving professional skills and taking advantage of career opportunities, individuals need to take time for relaxation and leisure. One cannot expect to work 60 hours per week and have time for family and friends. Rely on the time management and prioritization skills honed as a resident. Furthermore, remember to allow some time to give back to the profession. Serving on professional committees or task forces and volunteering in a free clinic are good ways to network and serve the profession. Likewise, be willing and enthusiastic about precepting and mentoring students and residents. Where would any pharmacist be today if not for their preceptors?

KEY POINTS

- Identify strengths to build on and weaknesses to correct.

- Begin the professional journey with a destination in mind, but be prepared for detours and roads of opportunity.

- Develop a list of ways (or a plan) to reach career goals.

- Develop a routine to stay current and cutting edge by committing to daily professional development.

- Find ways to give back to the profession.

REFERENCES

1. Rouse MJ. Continuing professional development in pharmacy. *Am J Health Syst Pharm.* 2004;61:2069–2076.
2. Board of Pharmacy Specialties. Specialties. http://www.bpsweb.org/specialties/pharmacotherapy.cfm. Accessed March 31, 2011.
3. Bostwick J, Howell H, Brady M. Beginning your career in academia at a new college of pharmacy. *Am J Health Syst Pharm.* 2008;65:1694–1698.

4. American Society of Health-System Pharmacists. CareerPharm. http://www
   .careerpharm.com. Accessed March 31, 2011.
5. American College of Clinical Pharmacy. Online position listings. http://www.accp.
   com/careers/onlinePositionListings.aspx. Accessed March 31, 2011.
6. White SJ, Tryon JE. How to find and succeed as a mentor. *Am J Health Syst
   Pharm.* 2007;64:1258–1259.
7. Pierpaoli PG. Mentors and residency training. *Am J Health Syst Pharm.*
   1990;47:112–113.

Index

Figures and tables are indicated by *f* and *t* following the page numbers.